An Introduction to Yoga

BESTSELLING NON-FICTION

- Abraham Lincoln by Lord Charnwood, ISBN: 9789380914251
- Annihilation of Caste by Dr B.R. Ambedkar, ISBN: 9789390492732
- Be What You Wish by Neville Goddard, ISBN: 9789387669550
- Civilization and Its Discontents by Sigmund Freud, ISBN: 9789387669499
- Guerrilla Warfare by Ernesto Che Guevara, ISBN: 9789354990366
- How I Made 2 Millions in the Stock Market by N. Darvas, ISBN: 9789389716283
- Jail Diary and Other Writings by Bhagat Singh, ISBN: 9789390492398
- Man-eaters of Kumaon by Jim Corbett, ISBN: 9789354990731
- My Experiments with Truth by Mahatma Gandhi, ISBN: 9789387669291
- Relativity by Albert Einstein, ISBN: 9789380914220
- Reminiscences of a Stock Operator by Edwin Lefevre, ISBN: 9788194764816
- Scientific Healing Affirmations by P. Yogananda, ISBN: 9789389716344
- Student's Encyclopedia of G.K. by Azeem Ahmad Khan, ISBN: 9789380914190
- The Art of War by Sun Tzu, ISBN: 9789380914893
- The Book of Five Rings by Miyamoto Musashi, ISBN: 9789354991202
- The Diary of a Young Girl by Anne Frank, ISBN: 9789380914312
- The Game of Life and How to Play It by F. Scovel Shinn, ISBN: 9789387669390
- The Law of Success by Napoleon Hill, ISBN: 9788180320927
- The Origin of Species by Charles Darwin, ISBN: 9788180320453
- The Power of Your Subconscious Mind by Joseph Murphy, ISBN: 9788180320958
- The Psychopathology of Everyday Life by Sigmund Freud, ISBN: 9789388118071
- The Richest Man in Babylon by George S. Clason, ISBN: 9789387669369
- The World as I See It by Albert Einstein, ISBN: 9789388118125
- Why I am an Atheist and Other Works by Bhagat Singh, ISBN: 9789354992162
- Zen in the Art of Archery by Eugen Herrigel, ISBN: 9789354991059

Search the book by its ISBN

An Introduction to

Yoga

ANNIE BESANT

GENERAL PRESS

Published by
GENERAL PRESS
4805/24, Fourth Floor, Krishna House
Ansari Road, Daryaganj, New Delhi - 110002
Ph : 011-23282971, 45795759
E-mail : generalpressindia@gmail.com

www.generalpress.in

First Edition : 2023

ISBN : 9789354995088

Published by Azeem Ahmad Khan for General Press

Contents

Foreword

These lectures are intended to give an outline of Yoga, in order to prepare the student to take up, for practical purposes, the Yoga sutras of Patanjali, the chief treatise on Yoga. I have on hand, with my friend Bhagavan Das as collaborateur, a translation of these Sutras, with Vyasa's commentary, and a further commentary and elucidation written in the light of Theosophy. To prepare the student for the mastering of that more difficult task, these lectures were designed; hence the many references to Patanjali. They may, however, also serve to give to the ordinary lay reader some idea of the Science of sciences, and perhaps to allure a few towards its study.

–Annie Besant

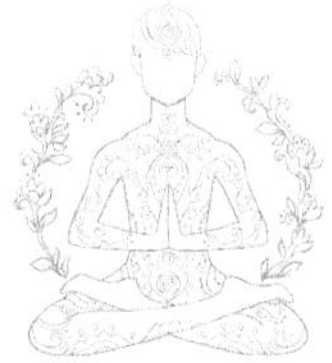

Lecture 1

The Nature of Yoga

In this first discourse we shall concern ourselves with the gaining of a general idea of the subject of Yoga, seeking its place in nature, its own character, its object in human evolution.

The Meaning of the Universe

Let us, first of all, ask ourselves, looking at the world around us, what it is that the history of the world signifies. When we read history, what does the history tell us? It seems to be a moving panorama of people and events, but it is really only a dance of shadows; the people are shadows, not realities, the kings and statesmen, the ministers and armies; and the events – the battles and revolutions, the rises and falls of states – are the most shadowlike dance of all. Even if the historian tries to go deeper, if he deals with economic conditions, with social organisations, with the study of the tendencies of the currents of thought, even then he is in the midst of shadows, the illusory shadows cast by unseen realities. This world is full of forms that are illusory, and the values are all wrong, the proportions are out of focus. The things which a man of the world thinks valuable, a spiritual man must cast aside as worthless. The diamonds of the world, with their glare and glitter in the rays of the outside sun, are mere fragments of broken glass to the man of knowledge. The crown of the king, the sceptre of the emperor, the triumph of earthly power, are less than nothing to the man who has had one glimpse of the majesty of the Self. What is, then, real? What is truly valuable? Our answer will be very different from the answer given by the man of the world.

"The universe exists for the sake of the Self." Not for what the outer world can give, not for control over the objects of desire, not for the sake even of beauty or pleasure, does the Great Architect plan and build His worlds. He has filled them with objects, beautiful and pleasure-giving. The great arch of the sky above, the mountains with snow-clad peaks, the valleys soft with verdure and fragrant with blossoms, the oceans with their vast depths, their surface now calm as a lake, now tossing in fury – they all exist, not for the objects themselves, but for their value to the Self. Not for themselves because they are anything in themselves but that the purpose of the Self may be served, and His manifestations made possible.

The world, with all its beauty, its happiness and suffering, its joys and pains" is planned with the utmost ingenuity, in order that the powers of the Self may be shown forth in manifestation. From the fire-mist to the LOGOS, all exist for the sake of the Self. The lowest grain of dust, the mightiest deva in his heavenly regions, the plant that grows out of sight in the nook of a mountain, the star that shines aloft over us-all these exist in order that the fragments of the one Self, embodied in countless forms, may realize their own identity, and manifest the powers of the Self through the matter that envelops them.

There is but one Self in the lowliest dust and the loftiest deva. "Mamamsaha" My portion, "a portion of My Self," says Sri Krishna, are all these Jivatmas, all these living spirits. For them the universe exists; for them the sun shines, and the waves roll, and the winds blow, and the rain falls, that the Self may know Himself as manifested in matter, as embodied in the universe.

The Unfolding of Consciousness

One of those pregnant and significant ideas which Theosophy scatters so lavishly around is this – that the same scale is repeated over and over again, the same succession of events in larger or smaller cycles. If you understand one cycle, you understand the whole. The same laws by which a solar system is builder go to the building up of the system of man. The laws by which the Self unfolds his powers in the universe, from the fire-mist up to the LOGOS, are the same laws of consciousness which repeat themselves in the universe of man. If you understand them in the one, you can equally understand them in the other. Grasp them in the small, and the large is revealed to you. Grasp them in the large, and the small becomes intelligible to you.

The great unfolding from the stone to the God goes on through millions of years, through aeons of time. But the long unfolding that takes place in the universe, takes place in a shorter time-cycle within the limit of humanity, and this in a cycle so brief that it seems as nothing beside the longer one. Within a still briefer cycle a similar unfolding takes place in the individual – rapidly, swiftly, with all the force of its past behind it. These forces that manifest and unveil themselves in evolution are cumulative in their power. Embodied in the stone, in the mineral world, they grow and put out a little more of strength, and in the mineral world accomplish their unfolding. Then they become too strong for the mineral, and press on into the vegetable world. There they unfold more and more of their divinity, until they become too mighty for the vegetable, and become animal.

Expanding within and gaining experiences from the animal, they again overflow the limits of the animal, and appear as the human. In the human being they still grow and accumulate with ever-increasing force, and exert greater pressure against the barrier; and then out of the human, they press into the super-human. This last process of evolution is called "Yoga."

Coming to the individual, the man of our own globe has behind him his long evolution in other chains than ours – this same evolution through mineral to vegetable, through vegetable to animal, through animal to man, and then from our last dwelling-place in the lunar orb on to this terrene globe that we call the earth. Our evolution here has all the force of the last evolution in it, and hence, when we come to this shortest cycle of evolution which is called Yoga, the man has behind him the whole of the forces accumulated in his human evolution, and it is the accumulation of these forces which enables him to make the passage so rapidly. We must connect our Yoga with the evolution of consciousness everywhere, else we shall not understand it at all; for the laws of evolution of consciousness in a universe are exactly the same as the laws of Yoga, and the principles whereby consciousness unfolds itself in the great evolution of humanity are the same principles that we take in Yoga and deliberately apply to the more rapid unfolding of our own consciousness. So that Yoga, when it is definitely begun, is not a new thing, as some people imagine.

The whole evolution is one in its essence. The succession is the same, the sequences identical. Whether you are thinking of the unfolding of consciousness in the universe, or in the human race, or in the individual, you can study the laws of the whole, and in Yoga you learn to apply those same laws to your own consciousness rationally and definitely. All the laws are one, however different in their stage of manifestation.

If you look at Yoga in this light, then this Yoga, which seemed so alien and so far off, will begin to wear a familiar face, and come to you in a garb not wholly strange. As you study the unfolding of consciousness, and the corresponding evolution of form, it will not seem so strange that from man you should pass on to superman, transcending the barrier of humanity, and finding yourself in the region where divinity becomes more manifest.

The Oneness of the Self

The Self in you is the same as the Self Universal. Whatever powers are manifested throughout the world, those powers exist in germ, in latency, in you. He, the Supreme, does not evolve. In Him there are no additions or subtractions. His portions, the Jivatmas, are as Himself, and they only unfold their powers in matter as conditions around them draw those powers forth. If you realize the unity of the Self amid the diversities of the Not-Self, then Yoga will not seem an impossible thing to you.

The Quickening of the Process of Self-unfoldment

Educated and thoughtful men and women you already are; already you have climbed up that long ladder which separates the present outer form of the Deity in you from His form in the dust. The manifest Deity sleeps in the mineral and the stone. He becomes more and more unfolded in vegetables and animals, and lastly in man He has reached what appears as His culmination to ordinary men. Having done so much, shall you not do more?

With the consciousness so far unfolded, does it seem impossible that it should unfold in the future into the Divine?

As you realize that the laws of the evolution of form and of the unfolding of consciousness in the universe and man are the same, and that it is through these laws that the yogi brings out his hidden powers, then you will understand also that it is not necessary to go into the mountain or into the desert, to hide yourself in a cave or a forest, in order that the union with the Self may be obtained – He who is within you and without you. Sometimes for a special purpose seclusion may be useful. It may be well at times to retire temporarily from the busy haunts of men. But in the universe planned by Isvara, in order that the powers of the Self may be brought out – there is your best field for Yoga, planned with Divine wisdom and sagacity. The world is meant for the unfolding of the Self: why should you then seek to run away from it? Look at Shri Krishna Himself in that great Upanishad of yoga, the Bhagavad-Gita. He spoke it out on a battle-field, and not on a mountain peak. He spoke it to a Kshattriya ready to fight, and not to a Brahmana quietly retired from the world. The Kurukshetra of the world is the field of Yoga. They who cannot face the world have not the strength to face the difficulties of Yoga practice. If the outer world out-wearies your powers, how do you expect to conquer the difficulties of the inner life? If you cannot climb over the little troubles of the world, how can you hope to climb over the difficulties that a yogi has to scale? Those men blunder, who think that running away from the world is the road to victory, and that peace can be found only in certain localities.

As a matter of fact, you have practised Yoga unconsciously in the past, even before your self- consciousness had separated itself, was aware of itself. Sand knew itself to be different, in temporary matter at least, from all the others that surround it. And that is the first idea that you should take up and hold firmly: Yoga is only a quickened process of the ordinary unfolding of consciousness.

Yoga may then be defined as the "rational application of the laws of the unfolding of consciousness in an individual case". That is what is meant by the methods of Yoga. You study the laws' of the unfolding of consciousness in the universe, you then apply them to a special case – and that case is your own. You cannot apply them to another. They must be self-applied. That is the definite principle to grasp. So we must add one more word to our definition: "Yoga is the rational application of the laws of the unfolding of consciousness, self-applied in an individual case."

Yoga is a Science

Next, Yoga is a science. That is the second thing to grasp. Yoga is a science, and not a vague, dreamy drifting or imagining. It is an applied science, a systematized collection of laws applied to bring about a definite end. It takes up the laws of psychology, applicable to the unfolding of the whole consciousness of man on every plane, in every world, and applies those rationally in a particular case. This rational application of the laws of unfolding consciousness acts exactly on the same principles that you see applied around you every day in other departments of science.

You know, by looking at the world around you, how enormously the intelligence of man, co-operating with nature, may quicken "natural" processes, and the working of intelligence is as "natural" as anything else. We make this distinction, and practically it is a real one, between "rational" and "natural" growth, because human intelligence can guide the working of natural laws; and when we come to deal with Yoga, we are in the same department of applied science as, let us say, is the scientific farmer or gardener, when he applies the natural laws of selection to breeding. The farmer or gardener cannot transcend the laws of nature, nor can he work against them. He has no other laws of nature to work with save universal laws by which nature is evolving forms around us, and yet he does in a few years what nature takes, perhaps, hundreds of thousands of years to do. And how? By applying human intelligence to choose the laws that serve him and to neutralize the laws that hinder. He brings the divine intelligence in man to utilise the divine powers in nature that are working for general rather than for particular ends.

Take the breeder of pigeons. Out of the blue rock pigeon he develops the pouter or the fan-tail; he chooses out, generation after generation, the forms that show most strongly the peculiarity that he wishes to develop. He mates such birds together, takes every favouring circumstance into consideration and selects again and again, and so on and on, till the peculiarity that he wants to establish has become a well-marked feature. Remove his controlling intelligence, leave the birds to themselves, and they revert to the ancestral type.

Or take the case of the gardener. Out of the wild rose of the hedge has been evolved every rose of the garden. Many-petalled roses are but the result of the scientific culture of the five-petalled rose of the hedgerow, the wild product of nature. A gardener who chooses the pollen from one plant and places it on the carpers of another is simply doing deliberately what is done every day by the bee and the fly. But he chooses his plants, and he chooses those that have the qualities he wants intensified, and from those again he chooses those that show the desired qualities still more clearly, until he has produced a flower so different from the original stock that only by tracing it back can you tell the stock whence it sprang.

So is it in the application of the laws of psychology that we call Yoga. Systematized knowledge of the unfolding of consciousness applied to the individualized Self, that is Yoga. As I have just said, it is by the world that consciousness has been unfolded, and the world is admirably planned by the LOGOS for this unfolding of consciousness; hence the would-be yogi, choosing out his objects and applying his laws, finds in the world exactly the things he wants to make his practice of Yoga real, a vital thing, a quickening process for the knowledge of the Self. There are many laws. You can choose those which you require, you can evade those you do not require, you can utilize those you need, and thus you can bring about the result that nature, without that application of human intelligence, cannot so swiftly effect.

Take it, then, that Yoga is within your reach, with your powers, and that even some of the lower practices of Yoga, some of the simpler applications of the laws of the unfolding of consciousness to yourself, will benefit you in this world as well as in all others. For you are really merely quickening your growth, your unfolding, taking advantage of the powers nature puts within your hands, and deliberately eliminating the conditions which would not help you in your work, but rather hinder your march forward. If you see it in that light, it seems to me that Yoga will be to you a far more real, practical thing, than it is when you merely read some fragments about it taken from Sanskrit books, and often mistranslated into English, and you will begin to feel that to be a yogi is not necessarily a thing for a life far off, an incarnation far removed from the present one.

Man a Duality

Some of the terms used in Yoga are necessarily to be known. For Yoga takes man for a special purpose and studies him for a special end and, therefore, only troubles itself about two great facts regarding man, mind and body. First, he is a unit, a unit of consciousness. That is a point to be definitely grasped. There is only one of him in each set of envelopes, and sometimes the Theosophist has to revise his ideas about man when he begins this practical line. Theosophy quite usefully and rightly, for the understanding of the human constitution, divides man into many parts and pieces. We talk of physical, astral, mental, etc. Or we talk about Sthula-sarira, Sukshma-sarira, Karana-sarira, and so on. Sometimes we divide man into Anna-maya-kosa, Prana-maya-kosa, Mano-maya-kosa, etc. We divide man into so many pieces in order to study him thoroughly, that we can hardly find the man because of the pieces. This is, so to say, for the study of human anatomy and physiology.

But Yoga is practical and psychological. I am not complaining of the various sub-divisions of other systems. They are necessary for the purpose of those systems. But Yoga, for its practical purposes, considers man simply as a duality – mind and body, a unit of consciousness in a set of envelopes. This is not the duality of the Self and the Not-Self. For in Yoga, "Self" includes consciousness plus such matter as it cannot distinguish from itself, and Not-Self is only the matter it can put aside.

Man is not pure Self, pure consciousness, Samvid. That is an abstraction. In the concrete universe there are always the Self and His sheaths, however tenuous the latter may be, so that a unit of consciousness is inseparable from matter, and a Jivatma, or Monad, is invariably consciousness plus matter.

In order that this may come out clearly, two terms are used in Yoga as constituting man, Prana and Pradhana, life-breath and matter. Prana is not only the life-breath of the body, but the totality of the life forces of the universe or, in other words, the life-side of the universe.

"I am Prana," says Indra. Prana here means the totality of the life-forces. They are taken as consciousness, mind. Pradhana is the term used for matter. Body, or the opposite of mind, means for the yogi in practice so much of the appropriated matter of the outer world as he is able to put away from himself, to distinguish from his own consciousness.

This division is very significant and useful, if you can catch clearly hold of the root idea. Of course, looking at the thing from beginning to end, you will see Prana, the great Life, the great Self, always present in all, and you will see the envelopes, the bodies, the sheaths, present at the different stages, taking different forms; but from the standpoint of yogic practice, that is called Prana, or Self, with which the man identifies himself for the time, including every sheath of matter from which the man is unable to separate himself in consciousness. That unit, to the yogi, is the Self, so that it is a changing quantity. As he drops off one sheath after another and says: "That is not myself," he is coming nearer and nearer to his highest point, to consciousness in a single film, in a single atom of matter, a Monad. For all practical purposes of Yoga, the man, the working, conscious man, is so much of him as he cannot separate from the matter enclosing him, or with which he is connected. Only that is body which the man is able to put aside and say: "This is not I, but mine." We find we have a whole series of terms in Yoga which may be repeated over and over again. All the states of mind exist on every plane, says Vyasa, and this way of dealing with man enables the same significant words, as we shall see in a moment, to be used over and over again, with an ever subtler connotation; they all become relative, and are equally true at each stage of evolution.

Now it is quite clear that, so far as many of us are concerned, the physical body is the only thing of which we can say: "It is not myself";

so that, in the practice of Yoga at first, for you, all the words that would be used in it to describe the states of consciousness, the states of mind, would deal with the waking consciousness in the body as the lowest state, and, rising up from that, all the words would be relative terms, implying a distinct and recognisable state of the mind in relation to that which is the lowest. In order to know how you shall begin to apply to yourselves the various terms used to describe the states of mind, you must carefully analyse your own consciousness, and find out how much of it is really consciousness, and how much is matter so closely appropriated that you cannot separate it from yourself.

States of Mind

Let us take it in detail. Four states of consciousness are spoken of amongst us. "Waking" consciousness or Jagrat; the "dream" consciousness, or Svapna; the "deep sleep" consciousness, or Sushupti; and the state beyond that, called Turiya[1] How are those related to the body?

Jagrat is the ordinary waking consciousness, that you and I are using at the present time. If our consciousness works in the subtle, or astral, body, and is able to impress its experiences upon the brain, it is called Svapna, or in English, dream consciousness; it is more vivid and real than the Jagrat state. When working in the subtler form – the mental body – it is not able to impress its experiences on the brain, it is called Sushupti or deep sleep consciousness; then the mind is working on its own contents, not on outer objects. But if it has so far separated itself from connection with the brain, that it cannot be readily recalled by outer means,

1. It is impossible to avoid the use of these technical terms, even in an introduction to Yoga. There are no exact English equivalents, and they are no more troublesome to learn than any other technical psychological terms.

then it is, called Turiya, a lofty state of trance. These four states, when correlated to the four planes, represent a much unfolded consciousness. Jagrat is related to the physical; Svapna to the astral; Sushupti to the mental; and Turiya to the Buddhist. When passing from one world to another, we should use these words to designate the consciousness working under the conditions of each world. But the same words are repeated in the books of Yoga with a different context. There the difficulty occurs, if we have not learned their relative nature. Svapna is not the same for all, nor is Sushupti the same for everyone.

Above all, the word Samadhi, to be explained in a moment, is used in different ways and in different senses. How then are we to find our way in this apparent tangle? By knowing the state which is the starting-point, and then the sequence will always be the same. All of you are familiar with the waking consciousness in the physical body. You can find four states even in that, if you analyse it, and a similar sequence of the states of the mind is found on every plane.

How to distinguish them, then? Let us take the waking consciousness, and try to see the four states in that. Suppose I take up a book and read it. I read the words; my eyes arc related to the outer physical consciousness. That is the Jagrat state. I go behind the words to the meaning of the words. I have passed from the waking state of the physical plane into the Svapna state of waking consciousness, that sees through the outer form, seeking the inner life. I pass from this to the mind of the writer; here the mind touches the mind; it is the waking consciousness in its Sushupti state. If I pass from this contact and enter the very mind of the writer, and live in that man's mind, then I have reached the Turiya state of the waking consciousness.

Take another illustration. I look at any watch; I am in Jagrat. I close my eyes and make an image of the watch; I am in Svapna. I call together many ideas of many watches, and reach the ideal watch; I am in Sushupti. I pass to the ideal of time in the abstract; I am in Turiya. But all these are stages in the physical plane consciousness; I have not left the body.

In this way, you can make states of mind intelligible and real, instead of mere words.

Samadhi

Some other important words, which recur from time to time in the Yoga-sutras, need to be understood, though there are no exact English equivalents. As they must be used to avoid clumsy circumlocutions, it is necessary to explain them. It is said: "Yoga is Samadhi." Samadhi is a state in which the consciousness is so dissociated from the body that the latter remains insensible. It is a state of trance in which the mind is fully self-conscious, though the body is insensitive, and from which the mind returns to the body with the experiences it has had in the super physical state, remembering them when again immersed in the physical brain. Samadhi for any one person is relative to his waking consciousness, but implies insensitiveness of the body. If an ordinary person throws himself into trance and is active on the astral plane, his Samadhi is on the astral. If his consciousness is functioning in the mental plane, Samadhi is there. The man who can so withdraw from the body as to leave it insensitive, while his mind is fully self-conscious, can practice Samadhi.

The phrase "Yoga is Samadhi" covers facts of the highest significance and greatest instruction. Suppose you are only able to reach the astral world when you are asleep, your consciousness there is, as we have seen, in the Svapna state. But as you slowly unfold your powers, the astral forms begin to intrude upon your waking physical consciousness until they appear as distinctly as do physical forms, and thus become objects of your waking consciousness. The astral world then, for you, no longer belongs to the Svapna consciousness, but to the Jagrat; you have taken two worlds within the scope of your Jagrat consciousness – the physical and the astral worlds – and the mental world is in your Svapna consciousness. "Your body" is then the physical and the astral bodies taken together. As you go on, the mental plane begins similarly to intrude itself, and the physical, astral and mental all come within your waking consciousness; all these are, then, your Jagrat world. These three worlds form but one world to you; their three corresponding bodies but one body, that perceives and acts. The three bodies of the ordinary man have become one body for the yogi. If under these conditions you want to see only one world at a time, you must fix your attention on it, and thus focus it. You can, in that state of enlarged waking, concentrate your attention on the physical and see it; then the astral and mental will appear hazy. So you can focus your attention on the astral and see it; then the physical and the mental, being out of focus, will appear dim. You will easily understand this if you remember that, in this hall, I may focus my sight in the middle of the hall, when the pillars on both sides will appear indistinctly. Or I may concentrate my attention on a pillar and see it distinctly, but I then see you only vaguely at the same time. It is a change of focus, not a change of body. Remember that all which you can put aside as not yourself is the body of the yogi, and hence, as you go higher, the lower bodies form but a single body and the consciousness in that sheath of matter which it still cannot throw away, that becomes the man.

"Yoga is Samadhi." It is the power to withdraw from all that you know as body, and to concentrate yourself within. That is Samadhi. No ordinary means will then call you back to the world that you have left.[1] This will also explain to you the phrase in The Secret Doctrine that the Adept "begins his Samadhi on the atomic plane" When a Jivan-Mukta enters into Samadhi, he begins it on the atomic plane. All planes below the atomic are one plane for him. He begins his Samadhi on a plane to which the mere man cannot rise. He begins it on the atomic plane, and thence rises stage by stage to the higher cosmic planes. The same word, Samadhi, is used to describe the states of the consciousness, whether it rises above the physical into the astral, as in self-induced trance of an ordinary man, or as in the case of a Jivan-Mukta when, the consciousness being already centred in the fifth, or atomic plane, it rises to the higher planes of a larger world.

The Literature of Yoga

Unfortunately for non-Sanskrit-knowing people, the literature of Yoga is not largely available in English. The general teachings of Yoga are to be found in the Upanishads, and the Bhagavad-Gita; those, in many translations, are within your reach, but they are general, not special; they give you the main principles, but do not tell you about the methods in any detailed way. Even in the Bhagavad-Gita, while you are told to make sacrifices, to become indifferent, and so on, it is all of the nature of moral precept, absolutely necessary indeed, but still not telling you how to reach the conditions put before you. The special literature of Yoga is, first of all, many of the minor Upanishads, "the hundred-and-eight"

1. An Indian yogi in Samadhi, discovered in a forest by some ignorant and brutal Englishmen, was so violently ill used that he returned to his tortured body, only to leave it again at once by death.

as they are called. Then comes the enormous mass of literature called the Tantras. These books have an evil significance in the ordinary English ear, but not quite rightly. The Tantras are very useful books, very valuable and instructive; all occult science is to be found in them. But they are divisible into three classes: those that deal with white magic, those that deal with black magic, and those that deal with what we may call grey magic, a mixture of the two. Now magic is the word which covers the methods of deliberately bringing about super-normal physical states by the action of the will.

A high tension of the nerves, brought on by anxiety or disease, leads to ordinary hysteria, emotional and foolish. A similarly high tension, brought about by the will, renders a man sensitive to super-physical vibrations Going to sleep has no significance, but going into Samadhi is a priceless power. The process is largely the same, but one is due to ordinary conditions, the other to the action of the trained will. The Yogi is the man who has learned the power of the will, and knows how to use it to bring about foreseen and fore determined results. This knowledge has ever been called magic; it is the name of the Great Science of the past, the one Science, to which only the word "great" was given in the past. The Tantras contain the whole of that; the occult side of man and nature, the means whereby discoveries may be made, the principles whereby the man may re-create himself, all these are in the Tantras. The difficulty is that without a teacher they are very dangerous, and again and again a man trying to practice the Tantric methods without a teacher makes himself very ill. So the Tantras have got a bad name both in the West and here in India. A good many of the American "occult" books now sold are scraps of the Tantras which have been translated. One difficulty is that these Tantric works often use the name of a bodily organ to represent an astral or mental centre. There is some reason in that because all the centres are connected with each other from body to body; but no reliable teacher would set his pupil to work on the bodily organs until he had some control over the higher centres, and had carefully purified the physical body. Knowing the one helps you to know the other, and the teacher who has been through it all can place his pupil on the right path; but it you take up these words, which are all physical, and do not know to what the physical word is applied, then you will only become very confused, and may injure yourself. For instance, in one of the Sutras it is said that if you meditate on a certain part of the tongue you will obtain astral sight. That means that if you meditate on the pituitary body, just over this part of the tongue, astral sight will be opened. The particular word used to refer to a centre has a correspondence in the physical body, and the word is often applied to the physical organs when the other is meant. This is what is called a "blind," and it is intended to keep the people away from dangerous practices in the books that are published; people may meditate on that part of their tongues all their lives without anything coming of it; but if they think upon the corresponding centre in the body, a good deal – much harm – may come of it. "Meditate on the navel," it is also said. This means the solar plexus, for there is a close connection between the two. But to meditate on that is to incur the danger of a serious nervous disorder, almost impossible to cure. All who know how many people in India suffer through these practices, ill-understood, recognize that it is not wise to plunge into them without someone to tell you what they mean, and what may be safely practiced and what not. The other part of the Yoga literature is a small book called the sutras of Patanjali. That is available, but I am afraid that few are able to make much of it by themselves. In the first place, to elucidate the Sutras, which are simply headings, there is a great deal of commentary in Sanskrit, only partially translated. And even the commentaries have this peculiarity, that all the most difficult words are merely repeated, not explained, so that the student is not much enlightened.

Some Definitions

There are a few words, constantly recurring, which need brief definitions, in order to avoid confusion; they are: Unfolding, Evolution, Spirituality, Psychism, Yoga and Mysticism.

"Unfolding" always refers to consciousness, "evolution" to forms. Evolution is the homogeneous becoming the heterogeneous, the simple becoming complex. But there is no growth and no perfectioning for Spirit, for consciousness; it is all there and always, and all that can happen to it is to turn itself outwards instead of remaining turned inwards. The God in you cannot evolve, but He may show forth His powers through matter that He has appropriated for the purpose, and the matter evolves to serve Him. He Himself only manifests what He is. And on that, many a saying of the great mystics may come to your mind: "Become," says St. Ambrose, "what you are"—a paradoxical phrase; but one that sums up a great truth: become in outer manifestation that which you are in inner reality. That is the object of the whole process of Yoga.

"Spirituality" is the realisation of the One. "Psychism" is the manifestation of intelligence through any material vehicle.[1]

"Yoga" is the seeking of union by the intellect, a science; "Mysticism" is the seeking of the same union by emotion.[2]

---

1. See London Lectures of 1907,"Spirituality and Psychism".
2. The word yoga may, of course, be rightly used of all union with the self, whatever the road taken. I am using it here in the narrower sense, as peculiarly connected with the intelligence, as a Science, herein following Patanjali.

See the mystic. He fixes his mind on the object of devotion; he loses self-consciousness, and passes into a rapture of love and adoration, leaving all external ideas, wrapped in the object of his love, and a great surge of emotion sweeps him up to God. He does not know how he has reached that lofty state. He is conscious only of God and his love for Him. Here is the rapture of the mystic, the triumph of the saint.

The yogi does not work like that. Step after step, he realises what he is doing. He works by science and not by emotion, so that any who do not care for science, finding it dull and dry, are not at present unfolding that part of their nature which will find its best help in the practice of Yoga. The yogi may use devotion as a means. This comes out very plainly in Patanjali. He has given many means whereby Yoga may be followed, and curiously, "devotion to Isvara" is one of several means. There comes out the spirit of the scientific thinker. Devotion to Isvara is not for him an end in itself, but means to an end – the concentration of the mind. You see there at once the difference of spirit. Devotion to Isvara is the path of the mystic. He attains communion by that. Devotion to Isvara as a means of concentrating the mind is the scientific way in which the yogi regards devotion. No number of words would have brought out the difference of spirit between Yoga and Mysticism as well as this. The one looks upon devotion to Isvara as a way of reaching the Beloved; the other looks upon it as a means of reaching concentration. To the mystic, God, in Himself is the object of search, delight in Him is the reason for approaching Him, union with Him in consciousness is his goal; but to the yogi, fixing the attention on God is merely an effective way of concentrating the mind. In the one, devotion is used to obtain an end; in the other, God is seen as the end and is reached directly by rapture.

God without and God Within

That leads us to the next point, the relation of God without to God within. To the yogi, who is the very type of Hindu thought, there is no definite proof of God save the witness of the Self within to His existence, and his idea of finding the proof of God is that you should strip away from your consciousness all limitations, and thus reach the stage where you have pure consciousness – save a veil of the thin nirvanic matter. Then you know that God is. So you read in the Upanishad: "Whose only proof is the witness of the Self." This is very different from Western methods of thought, which try to demonstrate God by a process of argument. The Hindu will tell you that you cannot demonstrate God by any argument or reasoning; He is above and beyond reasoning, and although the reason may guide you on the way, it will not prove to demonstration that God is. The only way you can know Him is by diving into yourself. There you will find Him, and know that He is without as well as within you; and Yoga is a system that enables you to get rid of everything from consciousness that is not God, save that one veil of the nirvanic atom, and so to know that God is, with an unshakable certainty of conviction. To the Hindu that inner conviction is the only thing worthy to be called faith, and this gives you the reason why faith is said to be beyond reason, and so is often confused with credulity. Faith is beyond reason, because it is the testimony of the Self to himself, that conviction of existence as Self, of which reason is only one of the outer manifestations; and the only true faith is that inner conviction, which no argument can either strengthen or weaken, of the innermost Self of you, that of which alone you are entirely sure. It is the aim of Yoga to enable you to reach that Self constantly not by a sudden glimpse of intuition, but steadily, unshakably, and unchangeably, and when that Self is reached, then the question: "Is there a God?" can never again come into the. human mind.

Changes of Consciousness and Vibrations of Matter

It is necessary to understand something about that consciousness which is your Self, and about the matter which is the envelope of consciousness, but which the Self so often identifies with himself. The great characteristic of consciousness is change, with a foundation of certainty that it is. The consciousness of existence never changes, but beyond this all is change, and only by the changes does consciousness become Self-consciousness. Consciousness is an ever changing thing, circling round one idea that never changes – Self-existence. The consciousness itself is not changed by any change of position or place. It only changes its states within itself.

In matter, every change of state is brought about by change of place. A change of consciousness is a change of a state; a change of matter is a change of place. Moreover, every change of state in consciousness is related to vibrations of matter in its vehicle. When matter is examined, we find three fundamental qualities – rhythm, mobility, stability – sattva, rajas, tamas. Sattva is rhythm, vibration. It is more than; rajas, or mobility. It is a regulated movement, a swinging from one side to the other over a definite distance, a length of wave, a vibration.

The question is often put: "How can things in such different categories, as matter and Spirit, affect each other? Can we bridge that great gulf which some say can never be crossed?" Yes, the Indian has crossed it, or rather, has shown that there is no gulf. To the Indian, matter and Spirit are not only the two phases of the One, but, by a subtle analysis of the relation between consciousness and matter, he sees that in every universe the LOGOS imposes upon matter a certain definite relation of rhythms, every vibration of matter corresponding to a change in consciousness. There is no change in consciousness, however subtle, that has not appropriated to it a vibration in matter; there is no vibration in matter, however swift or delicate, which has not correlated to it a certain change in consciousness. That is the first great work of the LOGOS, which the Hindu scriptures trace out in the building of the atom, the Tanmatra, "the measure of That," the measure of consciousness. He who is consciousness imposes on his material the answer to every change in consciousness, and that is an infinite number of vibrations. So that between the Self and his sheaths there is this invariable relation: the change in consciousness and the vibration of matter, and vice versa. That makes it possible for the Self to know the Not-Self.

These correspondences are utilised in Raja Yoga and Hatha Yoga, the Kingly Yoga and the Yoga of Resolve. The Raja Yoga seeks to control the changes in consciousness, and by this control to rule the material vehicles. The Hatha Yoga seeks to control the vibrations of matter, and by this control to evoke the desired changes in consciousness. The weak point in Hatha Yoga is that action on this line cannot reach beyond the astral plane, and the great strain imposed on the comparatively intractable matter of the physical plane sometimes leads to atrophy of the very organs, the activity of which is necessary for effecting the changes in consciousness that would be useful. The Hatha Yogi gains control over the bodily organs with which the waking consciousness no longer concerns itself, having relinquished them to its lower part, the "subconsciousness," This is often useful as regards the prevention of disease, but serves no higher purpose. When he begins to work on the brain centres connected with ordinary consciousness, and still more when he touches those connected with the super-consciousness, he enters a dangerous region, and is more likely to paralyse than to evolve.

That relation alone it is which makes matter cognizable; the change in the thinker is answered by a change outside, and his answer to it and the change in it that he makes by his answer re-arrange again the matter of the body which is his envelope. Hence the rhythmic changes in matter are rightly called its cognizability. Matter may be known by consciousness, because of this unchanging relation between the two sides of the manifest LOGOS who is one, and the Self becomes aware of changes within himself, and thus of those of the external words to which those changes are related.

Mind

What is mind? From the yogic standpoint it is simply the individualized consciousness, the whole of it, the whole of your consciousness including your activities which the Western psychologist puts outside mind. Only on the basis of Eastern psychology is Yoga possible. How shall we describe this individualized consciousness? First, it is aware of things. Becoming aware of them, it desires them. Desiring them, it tries to attain them. So we have the three aspects of consciousness – intelligence, desire, activity. On the physical plane, activity predominates, although desire and thought are present. On the astral plane, desire predominates, and thought and activity are subject to desire. On the mental plane; intelligence is the dominant note, desire and activity are subject to it. Go to the Buddhist plane, and cognition, as pure reason, predominates, and so on. Each quality is present all the time, but one predominates. So with the matter that belongs to them. In your combinations of matter you get rhythmic, active, or stable ones; and according to the combinations of matter in your bodies will be the conditions of the activity of the whole of these in consciousness. To practice Yoga you must build your bodies of the rhythmic combinations, with activity and inertia less apparent. The yogi wants to make his body match his mind.

Stages of Mind

The mind has five stages, Patanjali tells us, and Vyasa comments that "these stages of mind are on every plane". The first stage is the stage in which the mind is flung about, the Kshipta stage; it is the butterfly mind, the early stage of humanity, or, in man, the mind of the child, darting constantly from one object to another. It corresponds to activity on the physical plane. The next is the confused stage, Mudha, equivalent to the stage of the youth, swayed by emotions, bewildered by them; he begins to feel he is ignorant – a state beyond the fickleness of the child – a characteristic state, corresponding to activity in the astral world. Then comes the state of preoccupation, or infatuation, Vikshipta, the state of the man possessed by an idea – love, ambition, or what not. He is no longer a confused youth, but a man with a clear aim, and an idea possesses him. It may be either the fixed idea of the madman, or the fixed idea which makes the hero or the saint; but in any case he is possessed by the idea. The quality of the idea, its truth or falsehood, makes the difference between the maniac and the martyr.

Maniac or martyr, he is under the spell of a fixed idea. No reasoning avails against it. If he has assured himself that he is made of glass, no amount of argument will convince him to the contrary. He will always regard himself as being as brittle as glass. That is a fixed idea which is false. But there is a fixed idea which makes the hero and the martyr. For some great truth dearer than life is everything thrown aside. He is possessed by it, dominated by it, and he goes to death gladly for it. That state is said to be approaching Yoga, for such a man is becoming concentrated, even if only possessed by one idea. This stage corresponds to activity on the lower mental plane. Where the man possesses the idea, instead of being possessed by it, that one-pointed state of the mind, called Ekagrata in Sanskrit, is the fourth stage. He is a mature man, ready for the true life. When the man has gone through life dominated by one idea, then he is approaching Yoga; he is getting rid of the grip of the world, and is beyond its allurements. But when he possesses that which before possessed him, then he has become fit for Yoga, and begins the training which makes his progress rapid. This stage corresponds to activity on the higher mental plane.

Out of this fourth stage or Ekagrata, arises the fifth stage, Niruddha or Self-controlled. When the man not only possesses one idea but, rising above all ideas, chooses as he wills, takes or does not take according to the illumined Will, then he is Self-controlled and can effectively practice Yoga. This stage corresponds to activity on the Buddhist plane.

In the third stage, Vikshipta, where he is possessed by the idea, he is learning Viveka or discrimination between the outer and the inner, the real and the unreal. When he has learned the lesson of Viveka, then he advances a stage forward; and in Ekagrata he chooses one idea, the inner life; and as he fixes his mind on that idea he learns Vairagya or dispassion. He rises above the desire to possess objects of enjoyment, belonging either to this or any other world. Then he advances towards the fifth stage – Self-controlled. In order to reach that he must practice the six endowments, the Shatsamapatti. These six endowments have to do with the Will-aspect of consciousness as the other two, Viveka and Vairagya, have to do with the cognition and activity aspects of it.

By a study of your own mind, you can find out how far you are ready to begin the definite practice of Yoga. Examine your mind in order to recognize these stages in yourself. If you are in either of the two early stages, you are not ready for Yoga. The child and the youth are not ready to become yogis, nor is the preoccupied man. But if you find yourself possessed by a single thought, you are nearly ready for Yoga; it leads to the next stage of one-pointedness, where you can choose your idea, and cling to it of your own will. Short is the step from that to the complete control, which can inhibit all motions of the mind. Having reached that stage, it is comparatively easy to pass into Samadhi.

Inward and Outward-Turned Consciousness

Samadhi is of two kinds: one turned outward, one turned inward. The outward-turned consciousness is always first. You are in the stage of Samadhi belonging to the outward-turned waking consciousness, when you can pass beyond the objects to the principles which those objects manifest, when through the form you catch a glimpse of the life. Darwin was in this stage when he glimpsed the truth of evolution. That is the outward-turned Samadhi of the physical body.

This is technically the Samprajnata Samadhi, the "Samadhi with consciousness," but to be better regarded, I think, as with consciousness outward-turned, i.e. conscious of objects. When the object disappears, that is, when consciousness draws itself away from the sheath by which those objects are seen, then comes the Asamprajnata Samadhi; called the "Samadhi without consciousness". I prefer to call it the inward-turned consciousness, as it is by turning away from the outer that this stage is reached.

These two stages of Samadhi follow each other on every plane; the intense concentration on objects in the first stage, and the piercing thereby through the outer form to the underlying principle, are followed by the turning away of the consciousness from the sheath which has served its purpose, and its withdrawal into itself, i.e., into a sheath not yet recognised as a sheath. It is then for a while conscious only of itself and not of the outer world. Then comes the "cloud," the dawning sense again of an outer, a dim sensing of "something" other than itself; that again is followed by the functioning of the higher sheath and the Recognition of the objects of the next higher plane, corresponding to that sheath. Hence the complete cycle is: Samprajnata Samadhi, Asamprajnata Samadhi, Megha (cloud), and then the Samprajnata Samadhi of the next plane, and so on.

The Cloud

This term – in full, Dharma-Megha, cloud of righteousness, or of religion – is one which is very scantily explained by the commentators. In fact, the only explanation they give is that all the man's past karma of good gathers over him, and pours down upon him a rain of blessing. Let us see if we cannot find something more than this meagre interpretation.

The term "cloud" is very often used in mystic literature of the West; the "Cloud on the Mount," the "Cloud on the Sanctuary," the "Cloud on the Mercy-Seat," are expressions familiar to the student. And the experience which they indicate is familiar to all mystics in its lower phases, and to some in its fullness. In its lower phases, it is the experience just noted, where the withdrawal of the consciousness into a sheath not yet recognised as a sheath is followed by the beginning of the functioning of that sheath, the first indication of which is the dim sensing of an outer. You feel as though surrounded by a dense mist, conscious that you are not alone but unable to see. Be still; be patient; wait. Let your consciousness be in the attitude of suspense. Presently the cloud will thin, and first in glimpses, then in its full beauty, the vision of a higher plane will dawn on your entranced sight. This entrance into a higher plane will repeat itself again and again, until your consciousness, centred on the Buddhist plane and its splendouis having disappeared as your consciousness withdraws even from that exquisite sheath, you find yourself in the true cloud, the cloud on the sanctuary, the cloud that veils the Holiest, that hides the vision of the Self. Then comes what seems to be the draining away of the very life, the letting go of the last hold on the tangible, the hanging in a void, the horror of great darkness, loneliness unspeakable. Endure, endure. Everything must go. "Nothing out of the Eternal can help you." God only shines out in the stillness; as says the Hebrew: "Be still, and know that I am God." In that silence a Voice shall be heard, the voice of the Self, in that stillness a Life shall be felt, the life of the Self. In that void a Fullness shall be revealed, the fullness of the Self. In that darkness a Light shall be seen, the glory of the Self. The cloud shall vanish, and the shining of the Self shall be made manifest. That which was a glimpse of a far-off majesty shall become a perpetual realisation and, knowing the Self and your unity with it, you shall enter into the Peace that belongs to the Self alone.

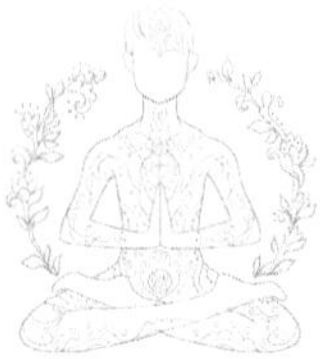

Lecture 2

Schools of Thought

In studying psychology anyone who is acquainted with the Sanskrit tongue must know how valuable that language is for precise and scientific dealing with the subject. The Sanskrit, or the well-made, the constructed, the built-together, tongue, is one that lends itself better than any other to the elucidation of psychological difficulties. Over and over again, by the mere form of a word, a hint is given, an explanation or relation is suggested. The language is constructed in a fashion which enables a large number of meanings to be connoted by a single word, so that you may trace all allied ideas, or truths, or facts, by this verbal connection, when you are speaking or using Sanskrit. It has a limited number of important roots, and then an immense number of words constructed on those roots.

Now the root of the word yoga is a word that means "to join," you, and that root appears in many languages, such as the English – of course, through the Latin, wherein you get jugare, jungere, "to join"—and out of that a number of English words are derived and will at once suggest themselves to you: junction, conjunction, disjunction, and so on. The English word "yoke" again, is derived from this same Sanskrit root so that all through the various words, or thoughts, or facts connected with this one root, you are able to gather the meaning of the word yoga and to see how much that word covers in the ordinary processes of the mind and how suggestive many of the words connected with it are, acting, so to speak, as sign-posts to direct you along the road to the meaning. In other tongues, as in French, we have a word like rapport, used constantly in English; "being en rapport," a French expression, but so Anglicized that it is continually heard amongst ourselves. And that term, in some ways, is the closest to the meaning of the Sanskrit word yoga; "to be in relation to"; "to be connected with"; "to enter into"; "to merge in"; and so on: all these ideas are classified together under the one head of "Yoga". When you find Sri Krishna saying that "Yoga is equilibrium," in the Sanskrit He is saying a perfectly obvious thing, because Yoga implies balance, yoking and the Sanskrit of equilibrium is "samvata – togetherness"; so that it is a perfectly simple, straightforward statement, not connoting anything very deep, but merely expressing one of the fundamental meanings of the word He is using. And so with another word, a word used in the commentary on the Sutra I quoted before, which conveys to the Hindu a perfectly straightforward meaning: "Yoga is Samadhi." To an only English-knowing person that does not convey any very definite idea; each word needs explanation. To a Sanskrit-knowing man the two words are obviously related to one another. For the word yoga, we have seen, means "yoked together," and Samadhi derived from the root dha, "to place," with the prepositions sam and a, meaning "completely together". Samadhi, therefore, literally means "fully placing together," and its etymological equivalent in English would be "to compose" (com=sam; posita=place).

Samadhi therefore means "composing the mind," collecting it together, checking all distractions. Thus by philological, as well as by practical, investigation the two words yoga and Samadhi are inseparably linked together. And when Vyasa, the commentator, says: "Yoga is the composed mind," he is conveying a clear and significant idea as to what is implied in Yoga. Although Samadhi has come to mean, by a natural sequence of ideas, the trance-state which results from perfect composure, its original meaning should not be lost sight of.

Thus, in explaining Yoga, one is often at a loss for the English equivalent of the manifold meanings of the Sanskrit tongue, and I earnestly advise those of you who can do so, at least to acquaint yourselves sufficiently with this admirable language, to make the literature of Yoga more intelligible to you than it can be to a person who is completely ignorant of Sanskrit.

It's Relation to Indian Philosophies

Let me ask you to think for a while on the place of Yoga in its relation to two of the great Hindu schools of philosophical thought, for neither the Westerner nor the non-Sanskrit-knowing Indian can ever really understand the translations of the chief Indian books, now current here and in the West, and the force of all the allusions they make, unless they acquaint themselves in some degree with the outlines of these great schools of philosophy, they being the very foundation on which these books are built up. Take the Bhagavad-Gita. Probably there are many who know that book fairly well, who use it as the book to help in the spiritual life, who are not familiar with most of its precepts. But you must always be more or less in a fog in reading it, unless you realise the fact that it is founded on a particular Indian philosophy and that the meaning of nearly all the technical words in it is practically limited by their meaning in philosophy known as the Samkhya. There are certain phrases belonging rather to the Vedanta, but the great majority are Samkhyan, and it is taken for granted that the people reading or using the book are familiar with the outline of the Samkhyan philosophy. I do not want to take you into details, but I must give you the leading ideas of the philosophy. For if you grasp these, you will not only read your Bhagavad-Gita with much more intelligence than before, but you will be able to use it practically for yogic purposes in a way that, without this knowledge, is almost impossible.

Alike in the Bhagavad-Gita and in the Yoga-sutras of Patanjali the terms are Samkhyan, and historically Yoga is based on the Samkhya, so far as its philosophy is concerned. Samkhya does not concern itself with, the existence of Deity, but only with the becoming of a universe, the order of evolution. Hence it is often called Nir-isvara Samkhya, the Samkhya without God. But so closely is it bound up with the Yoga system, that the latter is called Sesvara Samkhya, with God. For its understanding, therefore, I must outline part of the Samkhya philosophy, that part which deals with the relation of Spirit and matter; note the difference from this of the Vedantic conception of Self and Not-Self, and then find the reconciliation in the Theosophic statement of the facts in nature. The directions which fall from the lips of the Lord of Yoga in the Gita may sometimes seem to you opposed to each other and contradictory, because they sometimes are phrased in the Samkhyan and sometimes in the Vedantic terms, starting from different standpoints, one looking at the world from the standpoint of matter, the other from the standpoint of Spirit. If you are a student of Theosophy, then the knowledge of the facts will enable you to translate the different phrases. That reconciliation and understanding of these apparently contradictory phrases is the object to which I would ask your attention now.

The Samkhyan School starts with the statement that the universe consists of two factors, the first pair of opposites, Spirit and Matter, or more accurately Spirits and Matter. The Spirit is called Purusha – the Man; and each Spirit is an individual. Purusha is a unit, a unit of consciousness; they are all of the same nature, but distinct everlastingly the one from the other. Of these units there are many; countless Purushas are to be found in the world of men. But while they are countless in number they are identical in nature, they are homogeneous. Every Purusha has three characteristics, and these three are alike in all. One characteristic is awareness; it will become cognition. The second of the characteristics is life or prana; it will become activity. The third characteristic is immutability, the essence of eternity; it will become will. Eternity is not, as some mistakenly think, everlasting time. Everlasting time has nothing to do with eternity. Time and eternity are two altogether different things. Eternity is changeless, immutable, simultaneous. No succession in time, albeit everlasting – if such could be – could give eternity. The fact that Purusha has this attribute of immutability tells us that He is eternal; for changelessness is a mark of the eternal.

> *Such are the three attributes of Purusha, according to the Samkhya. Though these are not the same in nomenclature as the Vedantic Sat, Chit, Ananda, yet they are practically identical. Awareness or cognition is Chit; life or force is Sat; and immutability, the essence of eternity, is Ananda.*

Over against these Purushas, homogeneous units, countless in number, stands Prakriti, Matter, the second in the Samkhyan duality. Prakriti is one; Purushas are many. Prakriti is a continuum;

Purushas are discontinuous, being innumerable, homogeneous units. Continuity is the mark of Prakriti. Pause for a moment on the name Prakriti. Let us investigate its root meaning. The name indicates its essence. Pra means "forth," and kri is the root "make". Prakriti thus means "forth-making". Matter is that which enables the essence of Being to become. That which is Being – is-tence, becomes ex-is-tence – out being, by Matter, and to describe Matter as "forth-making" is to give its essence in a single word. Only by Prakriti can Spirit, or Purusha, "forth-make" or "manifest" himself. Without the presence of Prakriti, Purusha is helpless, a mere abstraction. Only by the presence of, and in Prakriti, can Purusha make manifest his powers. Prakriti has also three characteristics, the well-known gunas – attributes or qualities. These are rhythm, mobility and inertia. Rhythm enables awareness to become cognition. Mobility enables life to become activity. Inertia enables immutability to become will.

Now the conception as to the relation of Spirit to Matter is a very peculiar one, and confused ideas about it give rise to many misconceptions. If you grasp it, the Bhagavad-Gita becomes illuminated, and all the phrases about action and actor, and the mistake of saying "I act," become easy to understand, as implying technical Samkhyan ideas.

The three qualities of Prakriti, when Prakriti is thought of as away from Purusha, are in equilibrium, motionless, poised the one against the other, counter-balancing and neutralizing each other, so that Matter is called jada, unconscious, "dead". But in the presence of Purusha all is changed. When Purusha is in propinquity to Matter, then there is a change in Matter – not outside, but in it.

Purusha acts on Prakriti by propinquity, says Vyasa. It comes near Prakriti, and Prakriti begins to live. The "coming near" is a figure of speech, an adaptation to our ideas of time and space, for we cannot posit "nearness" of that which is timeless and space less – Spirit. By the word propinquity is indicated an influence exerted by Purusha on Prakriti, and this, where material objects are concerned, would be brought about by their propinquity. If a magnet be brought near to a piece of soft iron or an electrified body be brought near to a neutral one, certain changes are wrought in the soft iron or in the neutral body by that bringing near. The propinquity of the magnet makes the soft iron a magnet; the qualities of the magnet are produced in it, it manifests poles, it attracts steel, it attracts or repels the end of an electric needle. In the presence of a postively electrified body the electricity in a neutral body is re-arranged, and the positive retreats while the negative gathers near the electrified body. An internal change has occurred in both cases from the propinquity of another object. So with Purusha and Prakriti. Purusha does nothing, but from Purusha there comes out an influence, as in the case of the magnetic influence. The three gunas, under this influence of Purusha, undergo a marvellous change. I do not know what words to use, in order not to make a mistake in putting it. You cannot say that Prakriti absorbs the influence. You can hardly say that it reflects the Purusha. But the presence of Purusha brings about certain internal changes, causes a difference in the equilibrium of the three gunas in Prakriti. The three gunas were in a state of equilibrium. No guna was manifest. One guna was balanced against another. What happens when Purusha influences Prakriti? The quality of awareness in Purusha is taken up by, or reflected in, the guna called Sattva – rhythm, and it becomes cognition in Prakriti. The quality that we call life in Purusha is taken up by, or reflected, in the guna called Rajas – mobility, and it becomes force, energy, activity, in Prakriti. The quality that we call immutability in Purusha is taken up by, or reflected, in the guna called Tamas – inertia, and shows itself out as will or desire in Prakriti. So that, in that balanced equilibrium of Prakriti, a change has taken place by the mere propinquity of, or presence of, the Purusha. The Purusha has lost nothing, but at the same time a change has taken place in matter. Cognition has appeared in it. Activity, force, has appeared in it. Will or desire has appeared in it. With this change in Prakriti another change occurs. The three attributes of Purusha cannot be separated from each other, nor can the three attributes of Prakriti be separated each from each. Hence rhythm, while appropriating awareness, is under the influence of the whole three-in-one Purusha and cannot but also take up subordinately life and immutability as activity and will. And so with mobility and inertia. In combinations one quality or another may predominate, and we may have combinations which show preponderantly awareness-rhythm, or life-mobility, or immutability-inertia. The combinations in which awareness-rhythm or cognition predominates become "mind in nature," the subject or subjective half of nature. Combinations in which either of the other two predominates become the object or objective half of nature, the "force and matter" of the western scientist.[1]

We have thus nature divided into two, the subject and the object. We have now in nature everything that is wanted for the manifestation of activity, for the production of forms and for the expression of consciousness. We have mind, and we have force and matter. Purusha has nothing more to do, for he has infused all powers into Prakriti and sits apart, contemplating their interplay,

1. A friend notes that the first is the Suddha Sattva of the Ramanuja School, and the second and third the Prakriti, or spirit-matter, in the lower sense of the same.

himself remaining unchanged. The drama of existence is played out within Matter, and all that Spirit does is to look at it. Purusha is the spectator before whom the drama is played. He is not the actor, but only a spectator. The actor is the subjective part of nature, the mind, which is the reflection of awareness in rhythmic matter. That with which it works – objective nature, is the reflection of the other qualities of Purusha – life and immutability – in the gunas, Rajas and Tamas. Thus we have in nature everything that is wanted for the production of the universe. The Putusha only looks on when the drama is played before him. He is spectator, not actor. This is the predominant note of the Bhagavad-Gita. Nature does everything. The gunas bring about the universe. The man who says: "I act," is mistaken and confused; the gunas act, not he. He is only the spectator and looks on. Most of the Gita teaching is built upon this conception of the Samkhya, and unless that is clear in our minds we can never discriminate the meaning under the phrases of a particular philosophy.

Let us now turn to the Vedantic idea. According to the Vedantic view the Self is one, omnipresent, all-permeating, the one reality. Nothing exists except the Self – that is the starting-point in Vedanta. All permeating, all-controlling, all- inspiring, the Self is everywhere present. As the ether permeates all matter, so does the One Self permeate, restrain, support, vivify all. It is written in the Gita that as the air goes everywhere, so is the Self everywhere in the infinite diversity of objects. As we try to follow the outline of Vedantic thought, as we try to grasp this idea of the one universal Self, who is existence, consciousness, bliss, Sat-Chit-Ananda, we find that we are carried into a loftier region of philosophy than that occupied by the Samkhya. The Self is One. The Self is everywhere conscious, the Self is everywhere existent, the Self is everywhere blissful. There is no division between these qualities of the Self. Everywhere, all-embracing, these qualities are found at every point, in every place. There is no spot on which you can put your finger and say "The Self is not here." Where the Self is – and He is everywhere – there is existence, there is consciousness, and there is bliss. The Self, being consciousness, imagines limitation, division. From that imagination of limitation arises form, diversity, manyness. From that thought of the Self, from that thought of limitation, all diversity of the many is born. Matter is the limitation imposed upon the Self by His own will to limit Himself. "Eko'ham, bahu syam," "I am one; I will to the many"; "let me be many," is the thought of the One; and in that thought, the manifold universe comes into existence. In that limitation, Self-created, He exists, He is conscious, He is happy. In Him arises the thought that He is Self-existence, and behold! all existence becomes possible. Because in Him is the will to manifest, all manifestation at once comes into existence. Because in Him is all bliss, therefore is the law of life the seeking for happiness, the essential characteristic of every sentient creature. The universe appears by the Self-limitation in thought of the Self. The moment the Self ceases to think it, the universe is not, it vanishes as a dream. That is the fundamental idea of the Vedanta. Then it accepts the spirits of the Samkhya – the Purushas; but it says that these spirits are only reflections of the one Self, emanated by the activity of the Self and that they all reproduce Him in miniature, with the limitations which the universal Self has imposed upon them, which are apparently portions of the universe, but are really identical with Him. It is the play of the Supreme Self that makes the limitations, and thus reproduces within limitations the qualities of the Self; the consciousness of the Self, of the Supreme Self; becomes, in the particularised Self, cognition, the power to know; and the existence of the Self becomes activity, the power to manifest; and the bliss of the Self becomes will, the deepest part of all, the longing for happiness, for bliss; the resolve to obtain it is what we call will. And so in the limited, the power to know, and the power to act, and the power to will, these are the reflections in the particular Self of the essential qualities of the universal Self. Otherwise put: that which was universal awareness becomes now cognition in the separated Self; that which in the universal Self was awareness of itself becomes in the limited Self awareness of others; the awareness of the whole becomes the cognition of the individual. So with the existence of the Self: the Self-existence of the universal Self becomes, in the limited Self, activity, preservation of existence. So does the bliss of the universal Self, in the limited expression of the individual Self, become the will that seeks for happiness, the Self-determination of the Self, the seeking for Self-realisation, that deepest essence of human life.

The difference comes with limitation, with the narrowing of the universal qualities into the specific qualities of the limited Self; both are the same in essence, though seeming different in manifestation. We have the power to know, the power to will, and the power to act. These are the three great powers of the Self that show themselves in the separated Self in every diversity of forms, from the minutes organism to the loftiest Logos.

Then just as in the Samkhya, if the Purusha, the particular Self, should identify himself with the matter in which he is reflected, then there is delusion and bondage, so in the Vedanta, if the Self, eternally free, imagines himself to be bound by matter, identifying himself with his limitations, he is deluded, he is under the domain of Maya; for Maya is the self-identification of the Self with his limitations. The eternally free can never be bound by matter; the eternally pure can never be tainted by matter;

the eternally knowing can never be deluded by matter; the eternally Self-determined can never be ruled by matter, save by his own ignorance. His own foolish fancy limits his inherent powers; he is bound, because he imagines himself bound; he is impure, because he imagines himself impure; he is ignorant, because he imagines himself ignorant. With the vanishing of delusion he finds that he is eternally pure, eternally wise.

Here is the great difference between the Samkhya and the Vedanta. According to the Samkhya, Purusha is the spectator and never the actor. According to Vedanta the Self is the only actor, all else is maya: there is no one else who acts but the Self, according to the Vedanta teaching. As says the Upanishad: the Self willed to see, and there were eyes; the Self willed to hear, and there were ears; the Self willed to think, and there was mind. The eyes, the ears, the mind exist, because the Self has willed them into existence. The Self appropriates matter, in order that He may manifest His powers through it. There is the distinction between the Samkhya and the Vedanta: in the Samkhya the propinquity of the Purusha brings out in matter or Prakriti all these characteristics, the Prakriti acts and not the Purusha; in the Vedanta, Self alone exists and Self alone acts; He imagines limitation and matter appears; He appropriates that matter in order that He may manifest His own capacity.

The Samkhya is the view of the universe of the scientist: the Vedanta is the view of the universe of the metaphysician. Haeckel unconsciously expounded the Samkhyan philosophy almost perfectly. So close to the Samkhyan is his exposition, that another idea would make it purely Samkhyan; he has not yet supplied that propinquity of consciousness which the Samkhya postulates in its ultimate duality. He has Force and Matter, he has Mind in Matter, but he has no Purusha. His last book, criticised by

Sir Oliver Lodge, is thoroughly intelligible from the Hindu standpoint as an almost accurate representation of Samkhyan philosophy. It is the view of the scientist, indifferent to the "why" of the facts which he records. The Vedanta, as I said, is the view of the metaphysician he seeks the unity in which all diversities are rooted and into which they are resolved.

Now, what light does Theosophy throw on both these systems? Theosophy enables every thinker to reconcile the partial statements which are apparently so contradictory. Theosophy, with the Vedanta, proclaims the universal Self. All that the Vedanta says of the universal Self and the Self-limitation, Theosophy repeats. We call these Self-limited selves Monads, and we say, as the Vedantin says, that these Monads reproduce the nature of the universal Self whose portions they are. And hence you find in them the three qualities which you find in the Supreme. They are units' and these represent the Purushas of the Samkhya; but with a very great difference, for they are not passive watchers, but active agents in the drama of the universe, although, being above the fivefold universe, they are as spectators who pull the strings of the players of the stage. The Monad takes to himself from the universe of matter atoms which show out the qualities corresponding to his three qualities, and in these he thinks, and wills and acts. He takes to himself rhythmic combinations, and shows his quality of cognition. He takes to himself combinations that are mobile; through those he shows out his activity. He takes the combinations that are inert, and shows out his quality of bliss, as the will to be happy. Now notice the difference of phrase and thought. In the Samkhya, Matter changed to reflect the Spirit; in fact, the Spirit appropriates portions of Matter, and through those expresses his own characteristics – an enormous difference. He creates an actor for Self-expression, and this actor is the "spiritual man" of the Theosophical teaching, the spiritual Triad, the Atma-buddhi-manas, to whom we shall return in a moment.

The Monad remains ever beyond the fivefold universe, and in that sense is a spectator. He dwells beyond the five planes of matter. Beyond the Atomic, or Akasic; beyond the Buddhist plane, the plane of Vayu; beyond the mental plane, the plane of Agni; beyond the astral plane, the plane of Varuna; beyond the physical plane, the plane of Kubera. Beyond all these planes the Monad, the Self, stands Self-conscious and Self-determined. He reigns in changeless peace and lives in eternity. But as said above, he appropriates matter. He takes to himself an atom of the Atomic plane, and in that he, as it were, incorporates his will, and that becomes Atma. He appropriates an atom of the Buddhist plane, and reflects in that his aspect of cognition, and that becomes Buddha. He appropriates an atom of the manasic plane and embodies, as it were, his activity in it, and it becomes Manas. Thus we get Atma, plus Buddha, plus Manas. That triad is the reflection in the fivefold universe of the Monad beyond the fivefold universe. The terms of Theosophy can be easily identified with those of other schools. The Monad of Theosophy is the Jivatma of Indian philosophy, the Purusha of the Samkhya, the particularised Self of the Vedanta. The threefold manifestation, Atma-buddhi-manas, is the result of the Purusha's propinquity to Prakriti, the subject of the Samkhyan philosophy, the Self embodied in the highest sheaths, according to the Vedantic teaching. In the one you have this Self and His sheaths, and in the other the Subject, a reflection in matter of Purusha. Thus you can readily see that you are dealing with the same concepts but they are looked at from different standpoints. We are nearer to the Vedanta than to the Samkhya, but if you know the principles you can put the statements of the two philosophies in their own niches and will not be confused. Learn the principles and you can explain all the theories. That is the value of the Theosophical teaching; it gives you the principles and leaves you to study the philosophies, and you study them with a torch in your hand instead of in the dark.

Now when we understand the nature of the spiritual man, or Triad, what do we find with regard to all the manifestations of consciousness? That they are duads, Spirit-Matter everywhere, on every plane of our fivefold universe. If you are a scientist, you will call it spiritualised Matter; if you are a metaphysician you will call it materialised Spirit. Either phrase is equally true, so long as you remember that both are always present in every manifestation, that what you see is not the play of matter alone, but the play of Spirit-Matter, inseparable through the period of manifestation. Then, when you come, in reading an ancient book, to the statement "mind is material," you will not be confused; you will know that the writer is only speaking on the Samkhyan line, which speaks of Matter everywhere but always implies that the Spirit is looking on, and that this presence makes the work of Matter possible. You will not, when reading the constant statement in Indian philosophies that "mind is material," confuse this with the opposite view of the materialist which says that "mind is the product of matter"—a very different thing. Although the Samkhyan may use materialistic terms, he always posits the vivifying influence of Spirit, while the materialist makes Spirit the product of Matter. Really a gulf divides them, although the language they use may often be the same.

Mind

"Yoga is the inhibition of the functions of the mind," says Patanjali. The functions of the mind must be suppressed, and in order that we may be able to follow out really what this means, we must go more closely into what the Indian philosopher means by the word "mind".

Mind, in the wide sense of the term, has three great properties or qualities: cognition, desire or will, activity. Now Yoga is not immediately concerned with all these three, but only with one, cognition, the Samkhyan subject. But you cannot separate cognition, as we have seen, completely from the others, because consciousness is a unit, and although we are only concerned with that part of consciousness which we specifically call cognition, we cannot get cognition all by itself. Hence the Indian psychologist investigating this property, cognition, divides it up into three or, as the Vedanta says, into four (with all submission, the Vedantin here makes a mistake). If you take up any Vedantic book and read about mind, you will find a particular word used for it which. translated, means "internal organ". This Antah-Karana is the word always used where in English we use "mind"; but it is only used in relation to cognition, not in relation to activity and desire. It is said to be fourfold, being made up of Manas, Buddha, Ahamkara, and Chitta; but this fourfold division is a very curious division. We know what Manas is, what Buddha is, what Ahamkara is, but what is this Chitta? What is Chitta, outside Manas, Buddha and Ahamkara? Ask anyone you like. and record his answer; you will find that it is of the vaguest kind. Let us try to analyse it for ourselves, and see whether light will come upon it by using the Theosophic idea of a triplet summed up in a fourth, that is not really a fourth, but the summation of the three. Manas, Buddha and Ahamkara are the three different sides of a triangle,' which triangle is called Chitta. The Chitta is not a fourth, but the sum of the three: Manas, Buddha and Ahamkara. This is the old idea of a trinity in unity. Over and over again H. P. Blavatsky uses this summation as a fourth to her triplets, for she follows the old methods. The fourth, which sums up the three but is not other than they, makes a unity out of their apparent diversity. Let us apply that to Antahkarana.

Take cognition. Though in cognition that aspect of the Self is predominant, yet it cannot exist absolutely alone, The whole Self is there in every act of cognition. Similarly with the other two. One cannot exist separate from the others. Where there is cognition the other two are present, though subordinate to it. The activity is there, the will is there. Let us think of cognition as pure as it can be, turned on itself, reflected in itself, and we have Buddha, the pure reason, the very essence of cognition; this in the universe is represented by Vishnu, the sustaining wisdom of the universe. Now let us think of cognition looking outwards, and as reflecting itself in activity, its brother quality, and we have a mixture of cognition and activity which is called Manas, the active mind; cognition reflected in activity is Manas in man or Brahma, the creative mind, in the universe. When cognition similarly reflects itself in will, then it becomes Ahamkara, the "I am I" in man, represented by Mahadeva in the universe. Thus we have found within the limits of this cognition a triple division, making up the internal organ or Antahkarana – Manas, plus Buddha, plus Ahamkara – and we can find no fourth. What is then Chitta? It is the summation of the three, the three taken together, the totality of the three. Because of the old way of counting these things, you get this division of Antahkarana into four.

The Mental Body

We must now deal with the mental body, which is taken as equivalent to mind for practical purposes. The first thing for a man to do in practical Yoga is to separate himself from the mental body, to draw away from that into the sheath next above it. And here remember what I said previously, that in Yoga the Self is always the consciousness plus the vehicle from which the consciousness is unable to separate itself. All that is above the body you cannot leave is the Self for practical purposes, and your first attempt must be to draw away from your mental body. Under these conditions, Manas must be identified with the Self, and the spiritual Triad, the Atma-buddhi-manas, is to be realised as separate from the mental body. That is the first step. You must be able to take up and lay down your mind as you do a tool, before it is of any use to consider the further progress of the Self in getting rid of its envelopes. Hence the mental body is taken as the starting point. Suppress thought. Quiet it. Still it. Now what is the ordinary condition of the mental body? As you look upon that body from a higher plane, you see constant changes of colours playing in it. You find that they are sometimes initiated from within, sometimes from without. Sometimes a vibration from without has caused a change in consciousness, and a corresponding change in the colours in the mental body. If there is a change of consciousness, that causes vibration in the matter in which that consciousness is functioning. The mental body is a body of ever-changing hues and colours, never still, changing colour with swift rapidity throughout the whole of it. Yoga is the stopping of all these, the inhibition of vibrations and changes alike. Inhibition of the change of consciousness stops the vibration of the mental body; the checking of the vibration of the mental body checks the change in consciousness. In the mental body of a Master there is no change of colour save as initiated from within; no outward stimulus can produce any answer, any vibration, in that perfectly controlled mental body. The colour of the mental body of a Master is as moonlight on the rippling ocean. Within that whiteness of moon-like refulgence lie all possibilities of colour, but nothing in the outer world can make the faintest change of hue sweep over its steady radiance. If a change of consciousness occurs within, then the change will send a wave of delicate hues over the mental body which responds only in colour to changes initiated from within and never to changes stimulated from without. His mental body is never His Self, but only His tool or instrument, which He can take up or lay down at His will. It is only an outer sheath that He uses when He needs to communicate with the lower world.

By that idea of the stopping of all changes of colour in the mental body you can realise what is meant by inhibition. The functions of mind are stopped in Yoga. You have to begin with your mental body. You have to learn how to stop the whole of those vibrations, how to make the mental body colourless, still and quiet, responsive only to the impulses that you choose to put upon it. How will you be able to tell when the mind is really coming under control, when it is no longer a part of your Self? You will begin to realise this when you find that, by the action of your will, you can check the current of thought and hold the mind in perfect stillness. Sheath after sheath has to be transcended, and the proof of transcending is that it can no longer affect you. You can affect it, but it cannot affect you. The moment that nothing outside you can harass you, can stir the mind, the moment that the mind does not respond to the outer, save under your own impulse, then can you say of it: "This is not my Self." It has become part of the outer, it can no longer be identified with the Self.

From this you pass on to the conquest of the causal body in a similar way. When the conquering of the causal body is complete then you go to the conquering of the Buddhist body. When mastery over the Buddhist body is complete, you pass on to the conquest of the Atomic body.

Mind and Self

You cannot be surprised that under these conditions of continued disappearance of functions, the unfortunate student asks: "What becomes of the mind itself? If you suppress all the functions, what is left?" In the Indian way of teaching, when you come to a difficulty, someone jumps up and asks a question. And in the commentaries, the question which raises the difficulty is always put. The answer of Patanjali is: "Then the spectator remains in his own form." Theosophy answers: "The Monad remains." It is the end of the human pilgrimage. That is the highest point to which humanity may climb: to suppress all the reflections in the fivefold universe through which the Monad has manifested his powers, and then for the Monad to realise himself, enriched by the experiences through which his manifested aspects have passed. But to the Samkhyan the difficulty is very great, for when he has only his spectator left, when spectacle ceases, the spectator himself almost vanishes. His only function was to look on at the play of mind. When the play of mind is gone, what is left? He can no longer be a spectator, since there is nothing to see. The only answer is: "He remains in his own form." He is now out of manifestation, the duality is transcended, and so the Spirit sinks back into latency, no longer capable of manifestation. There you come to a very serious difference with the Theosophical view of the universe, for according to that view of the universe, when all these functions have been suppressed, then the Monad is ruler over matter and is prepared for a new cycle of activity, no longer slave but master.

All analogy shows us that as the Self withdraws from sheath after sheath, he does not lose but gains in Self-realisation. Self-realisation becomes more and more vivid with each successive withdrawal; so that as the Self puts aside one veil of matter after another, recognises in regular succession that each body in turn is not himself, by that process of withdrawal his sense of Self-reality becomes keener, not less keen. It is important to remember that, because often Western readers, dealing with Eastern ideas, in consequence of misunderstanding the meaning of the state of liberation, or the condition of Nirvana, identify it with nothingness or unconsciousness – an entirely mistaken idea which is apt to colour the whole of their thought when dealing with Yogic processes. Imagine the condition of a man who identifies himself completely with the body, so that he cannot, even in thought, separate himself from it – the state of the early undeveloped man – and compare that with the strength, vigour and lucidity of your own mental consciousness.

The consciousness of the early man limited to the physical body, with occasional touches of dream consciousness, is very restricted in its range. He has no idea of the sweep of your consciousness, of your abstract thinking. But is that consciousness of the early man more vivid, or less vivid, than yours? Certainly you will say, it is less vivid. You have largely transcended his powers of consciousness. Your consciousness is astral rather than physical, but has thereby increased its vividness. As the Self withdraws himself from sheath after sheath, he realises himself more and more, not less and less; Self-realisation becomes more intense, as sheath after sheath is cast aside. The centre grows more powerful as the circumference becomes more permeable, and at last a stage is reached when the centre knows itself at every point of the circumference. When that is accomplished the circumference vanishes, but not so the centre. The centre still remains. Just as you are more vividly conscious than the early man, just as your consciousness is more alive, not less, than that of an undeveloped man, so it is as we climb up the stairway of life and cast away garment after garment. We become more conscious of existence, more conscious of knowledge, more conscious of Self-determined power. The faculties of the Self shine out more strongly, as veil after veil falls away. By analogy, then, when we touch the Monad, our consciousness should be mightier, more vivid, and more perfect. As you learn to truly live, your powers and feelings grow in strength.

And remember that all control is exercised over sheaths, over portions of the Not-Self. You do not control your Self; that is a misconception; you control your Not-Self. The Self is never controlled; He is the Inner Ruler Immortal. He is the controller, not the controlled. As sheath after sheath becomes subject to your Self, and body after body becomes the tool of your Self, then shall you realise the truth of the saying of the Upanishad, that you are the Self, the Inner Ruler, the immortal.

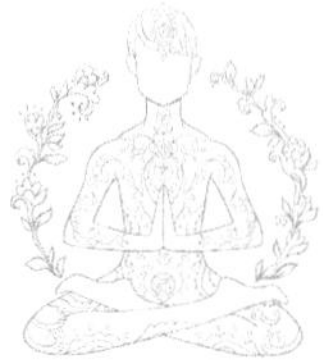

Lecture 3

Yoga as Science

I propose now to deal first with the two great methods of Yoga, one related to the Self and the other to the Not-Self. Let me remind you, before I begin, that we are dealing only with the science of Yoga and not with other means of attaining union with the Divine. The scientific method, following the old Indian conception, is the one to which I am asking your attention. I would remind you, however, that, though I am only dealing with this, there remain also the other two great ways of Bhakti and Karma. The Yoga we are studying specially concerns the Marga of Jnanam or knowledge, and within that way, within that Marga or path of knowledge, we find that three subdivisions occur, as everywhere in nature.

Methods of Yoga

With regard to what I have just called the two great methods in Yoga, we find that by one of these a man treads the path of knowledge by Buddha – the pure reason; and the other the same path by Manas – the concrete mind. You may remember that in speaking yesterday of the sub- divisions of Antah-karana, I pointed out to you that there we had a process of reflection of one quality in another; and within the limits of the cognitional aspect of the Self, you find Buddha, cognition reflected in cognition; and Ahamkara, cognition reflected in will; and Manas, cognition reflected in activity. Bearing those three sub-divisions in mind, you will very readily be able to see that these two methods of Yoga fall naturally under two of these heads. But what of the third? What of the will, of which Ahamkara is the representative in cognition? That certainly has its road, but it can scarcely be said to be a "method". Will breaks its way upwards by sheer unflinching determination, keeping its eyes fixed on the end, and using either Buddha or manes indifferently as a means to that end. Metaphysics is used to realise the Self; science is used to understand the Not-Self; but either is grasped, either is thrown aside, as it serves, or fails to serve, the needs of the moment. Often the man, in whom will is predominant, does not know how he gains the object he is aiming at; it comes to his hands, but the "how" is obscure to him; he willed to have it, and nature gives it to him. This is also seen in Yoga in the man of Ahamkara, the sub-type of will in cognition. Just as in the man of Ahamkara, Buddha and Manas are subordinate, so in the man of Buddha, Ahamkara and Manas are not absent, but are subordinate; and in the man of Manas, Ahamkara and Buddha are present, but play a subsidiary part. Both the metaphysician and the scientist must be supported by Ahamkara. That Self-determining faculty, that deliberate setting of oneself to a chosen end, that is necessary in all forms of Yoga. Whether a Yogi is going to follow the purely cognitional way of Buddha, or whether he is going to follow the more active path of Manas, in both cases he needs the self-determining will in order to sustain him in his arduous task. You remember it is written in the Upanishad that the weak man cannot reach the Self. Strength is wanted. Determination is wanted. Perseverance is wanted. And you must have, in every successful Yogi, that intense determination which is the very essence of individuality.

Now what are these two great methods? One of them may be described as seeking the Self by the Self; the other may be described as seeking the Self by the Not-Self; and if you will think of them in that fashion, I think you will find the idea illuminative. Those who seek the Self by the Self, seek him through the faculty of Buddha; they turn ever inwards, and turn away from the outer world. Those who seek the Self by the Not-Self, seek him through the active working Manas; they are outward-turned, and by study of the Not-Self, they learn to realise the Self. The one is the path of the metaphysician; the other is the path of the scientist.

To the Self by the Self

Let us look at this a little more closely, with its appropriate methods. The path on which the faculty of Buddha is used predominantly is, as just said, the path of the metaphysician. It is the path of the philosopher. He turns inwards, ever seeking to find the Self by diving into the recesses of his own nature. Knowing that the Self is within him, he tries to strip away vesture after vesture, envelope after envelope, and by a process of rejecting them he reaches the glory of the unveiled Self. To begin this, he must give up concrete thinking and dwell amidst abstractions. His method, then, must be strenuous, long-sustained, patient meditation. Nothing else will serve his end; strenuous, hard thinking, by which he rises away from the concrete into the abstract regions of the mind; strenuous, hard thinking, further continued, by which he reaches from the abstract region of the mind up to the region of Buddha, where unity is sensed; still by strenuous thinking, climbing yet further, until Buddha as it were opens out into Atma, until the Self is seen in his splendour, with only a film of atomic matter, the envelope of Atma in the manifested fivefold world. It is along that difficult and strenuous path that the Self must be found by way of the Self.

Such a man must utterly disregard the Not-Self. He must shut his senses against the outside world. The world must no longer be able to touch him. The senses must be closed against all the vibrations that come from without, and he must turn a deaf ear, a blind eye, to all the allurements of matter, to all the diversity of objects, which make up the universe of the Not-Self. Seclusion will help him, until he is strong enough to close himself against the outer stimuli or allurements. The contemplative orders in the Roman Catholic Church offer a good environment for this path. They put the outer world away, as far away as possible. It is a snare, a temptation, a hindrance. Always turning away from the world, the Yogi must fix his thought, his attention, upon the Self. Hence for those who walk along this road, what are called the Siddhis are direct obstacles, and not helps. But that statement that you find so often, that the Siddhis are things to be avoided, is far more sweeping than some of our modern Theosophists are apt to imagine. They declare that the Siddhis are to be avoided, but forget that the Indian who says this also avoids the use of the physical senses. He closes physical eyes and ears as hindrances. But some Theosophists urge avoidance of all use of the astral senses and mental senses, but they do not object to the free use of the physical senses, or dream that they are hindrances. Why not? If the senses are obstacles in their finer forms, they are also obstacles in their grosser manifestations. To the man who would find the Self by the Self, every sense is a hindrance and an obstacle, and there is no logic, no reason, in denouncing the subtler senses only, while forgetting the temptations of the physical senses, impediments as much as the other. No such division exists for the man who tries to understand the universe in which he is. In the search for the Self by the Self, all that is not Self is an obstacle. Your eyes, your ears, everything that puts you into contact with the outer world, is just as much an obstacle as the subtler forms of the same senses which put you into touch with the subtler worlds of matter, which you call astral and mental. This exaggerated fear of the Siddhis is only a passing reaction, not based on understanding but on lack of understanding; and those who denounce the Siddhis should rise to the logical position of the Hindu Yogi, or of the Roman Catholic recluse, who denounces all the senses, and all the objects of the senses, as obstacles in the way. Many Theosophists here, and more in the West, think that much is gained by acuteness of the physical senses, and of the other faculties in the physical brain; but the moment the senses are acute enough to be astral, or the faculties begin to work in astral matter, they treat them as objects of denunciation. That is not rational. It is not logical. Obstacles, then, are all the senses, whether you call them Siddhis or not, in the search for the Self by turning away from the Not-Self.

It is necessary for the man who seeks the Self by the Self to have the quality which is called "faith," in the sense in which I defined it before – the profound, intense conviction, that nothing can shake, of the reality of the Self within you. That is the one thing that is worthy to be dignified by the name of faith. Truly it is beyond reason, for not by reason may the Self be known as real. Truly it is not based on argument, for not by reasoning may the Self be discovered. It is the witness of the Self within you to his own supreme reality, and that unshakable conviction, which is shraddha, is necessary for the treading of this path. It is necessary, because without it the human mind would fail, the human courage would be daunted, the human perseverance would break, with the difficulties of the seeking for the Self. Only that imperious conviction that the Self is, only that can cheer the pilgrim in the darkness that comes down upon him, in the void that he must cross before – the life of the lower being thrown away – the life of the higher is realised. This imperious faith is to the Yogi on this path what experience and knowledge are to the Yogi on the other.

To the Self through the Not-self

Turn from him to the seeker for the Self through the Not- Self. This is the way of the scientist, of the man who uses the concrete, active Manas, in order scientifically to understand the universe; he has to find the real among the unreal, the eternal among the changing, the Self amid the diversity of forms. How is he to do it? By a close and rigorous study of every changing form in which the Self has veiled himself. By studying the Not-Self around him and in him, by understanding his own nature, by analysing in order to understand, by studying nature in others as well as in himself, by learning to know himself and to gain knowledge of others; slowly, gradually, step by step, plane after plane, he has to climb upwards, rejecting one form of matter after another, finding not in these the Self he seeks. As he learns to conquer the physical plane, he uses the keenest senses in order to understand, and finally to reject. He says: "This is not my Self. This changing panorama, these obscurities, these continual transformations, these are obviously the antithesis of the eternity, the lucidity, the stability of the Self. These cannot be my Self." And thus he constantly rejects them. He climbs on to the astral plane and, using there the finer astral senses, he studies the astral world, only to find that that also is changing and manifests not the changelessness of the Self. After the astral world is conquered and rejected, he climbs on into the mental plane, and there still studies the ever-changing forms of that Manasic world, only once more to reject them: "These are not the Self." Climbing still higher, ever following the track of forms, he goes from the mental to the Buddhist plane, where the Self begins to show his radiance and beauty in manifested union. Thus by studying diversity he reaches the conception of unity, and is led into the understanding of the One. To him the realisation of the Self comes through the study of the Not-Self, by the separation of the Not-Self from the Self. Thus he does by knowledge and experience what the other does by pure thinking and by faith. In this path of finding the Self through the Not-Self, the so-called Siddhis are necessary. Just as you cannot study the physical world without the physical senses, so you cannot study the astral world without the astral senses, nor the mental world without the mental senses. Therefore, calmly choose your ends, and then think out your means, and you will not be in any difficulty about the method you should employ, the path you should tread.

Thus we see that there are two methods, and these must be kept separate in your thought. Along the line of pure thinking – the metaphysical line – you may reach the Self. So also along the line of scientific observation and experiment – the physical line, in the widest sense of the term physical – you may reach the Self. Both are ways of Yoga. Both are included in the directions that you may read in the Yoga Sutras of Patanjali. Those directions will cease to be self-contradictory, if you will only separate in your thought the two methods. Patanjali has given, in the later part of his Sutras, some hints as to the way in which the Siddhis may be developed. Thus you may find your way to the Supreme.

Yoga and Morality

The next point that I would pause upon, and ask you to realise, is the fact that Yoga is a science of psychology. I want further to point out to you that it is not a science of ethic, though ethic is certainly the foundation of it. Psychology and ethic are not the same. The science of psychology is the result of the study of mind. The science of ethic is the result of the study of conduct, so as to bring about the harmonious relation of one to another. Ethic is a science of life, and not an investigation into the nature of mind and the methods by which the powers of the mind may be developed and evolved. I pause on this because of the confusion that exists in many people as regards this point. If you understand the scope of Yoga aright, such a confusion ought not to arise. The confused idea makes people think that in Yoga they ought to find necessarily what are called precepts of morality, ethic. Though Patanjali gives the universal precepts of morality and right conduct in the first two angas of Yoga, called yama and niyama, yet they are subsidiary to the main topic, are the foundation of it, as just said. No practice of Yoga is possible unless you possess the ordinary moral attributes summed up in yama and niyama; that goes without saying. But you should not expect to find moral precepts in a scientific text book of psychology, like Yoga. A man studying the science of electricity is not shocked if he does not find in it moral precepts; why then should one studying Yoga, as a science of psychology, expect to find moral precepts in it? I do not say that morality is unimportant for the Yogi. On the contrary, it is all-important. It is absolutely necessary in the first stages of Yoga for everyone. But to a Yogi who has mastered these, it is not necessary, if he wants to follow the left-hand path. For you must remember that there is a Yoga of the left-hand path, as well as a Yoga of the right-hand path. Yoga is there also followed, and though asceticism is always found in the early stages, and sometimes in the later, true morality is absent. The black magician is often as rigid in his morality as any Brother of the White Lodge.[1] Of the disciples of the black and white magicians, the disciple of the black magician is often the more ascetic. His object is not the purification of life for the sake of humanity, but the purification of the vehicle, that he may be better able to acquire power. The difference between the white and the black magician lies in the motive. You might have a white magician, a follower of the right-hand path, rejecting meat because the way of obtaining it is against the law of compassion. The follower of the left-hand path may also reject meat, but for the reason that he would not be able to work so well with his vehicle if it were full of the rajasic elements of meat. The difference is in the motive. The outer action is the same. Both men may be called moral, if judged by the outer action alone. The motive marks the path, while the outer actions are often identical.

It is a moral thing to abstain from meat, because thereby you are lessening the infliction of suffering; it is not a moral act to abstain from meat from the yogic standpoint, but only a means to an end. Some of the greatest yogis in Hindu literature were, and are, men whom you would rightly call black magicians. But still they are yogis. One of the greatest yogis of all was Ravana, the anti-Christ, the Avatara of evil, who summed up all the evil of the world in his own person in order to oppose the Avatara of good. He was a great, a marvellous yogi, and by Yoga he gained

1. Terms while and black as used here have no relation to race or colour.

his power. Ravana was a typical yogi of the left-hand path, a great destroyer, and he practiced Yoga to obtain the power of destruction, in order to force from the hands of the Planetary Logos the boon that no man should be able to kill him. You may say: "What a strange thing that a man can force from God such a power." The laws of Nature are the expression of Divinity, and if a man follows a law of Nature, he reaps the result which that law inevitably brings; the question whether he is good or bad to his fellow men does not touch this matter at all. Whether some other law is or is not obeyed, is entirely outside the question. It is a matter of dry fact that the scientific man may be moral or immoral, provided that his immorality does not upset his eyesight or nervous system. It is the same with Yoga. Morality matters profoundly, but it does not affect these particular things, and if you think it does, you are always getting into bogs and changing your moral standpoint, either lowering or making it absurd. Try to understand; that is what the Theosophist should do; and when you understand, you will not fall into the blunders nor suffer the bewilderment many do, when you expect laws belonging to one region of the universe to bring about results in another. The scientific man understands that. He knows that a discovery in chemistry does not depend upon his morality, and he would not think of doing an act of charity with a view to finding out a new element. He will not fail in a well-wrought experiment, however vicious his private life may be. The things are in different regions, and he does not confuse the laws of the two. As Ishvara is absolutely just, the man who obeys a law reaps the fruit of that law, whether his actions, in any other fields, are beneficial to man or not. If you sow rice, you will reap rice; if you sow weeds, you will reap weeds; rice for rice, and weed for weed. The harvest is according to the sowing. For this is a universe of law. By law we conquer, by law we succeed. Where does morality come in, then? When you are dealing with a magician of the right-hand path, the servant of the White Lodge, there morality is an all-important factor. Inasmuch as he is learning to be a servant of humanity, he must observe the highest morality, not merely the morality of the world, for the white magician has to deal with helping on harmonious relations between man and man. The white magician must be patient. The black magician may quite well be harsh. The white magician must be compassionate; compassion widens out his nature, and he is trying to make his consciousness include the whole of humanity. But not so the black magician. He can afford to ignore compassion.

A white magician may strive for power. But when he is striving for power, he seeks it that he may serve humanity and become more useful to mankind, a more effective servant in the helping of the world. But not so the brother of the dark side. When he strives for power, he seeks if for himself, so that he may use it against the whole world. He may be harsh and cruel. He wants to be isolated; and harshness and cruelty tend to isolate him. He wants power; and holding that power for himself, he can put himself temporarily, as it were, against the Divine Will in evolution.

The end of the one is Nirvana, where all separation has ceased. The end of the other is Avichi – the uttermost isolation – the kaivalya of the black magician. Both are yogis, both follow the science of yoga, and each gets the result of the law he has followed: one the kaivalya of Nirvana, the other the kaivalya of Avichi.

Composition of States of the Mind

Let us pass now to the "states of the mind" as they are called. The word which is used for the states of the mind by Patanjali is Vritti. This admirably constructed language Sanskrit gives you in that very word its own meaning. Vrittis means the "being" of the mind; the ways in which mind can exist; the modes of the mind; the modes of mental existence; the ways of existing. That is the literal meaning of this word. A subsidiary meaning is a "turning around," a "moving in a circle". You have to stop, in Yoga, every mode of existing in which the mind manifests itself. In order to guide you towards the power of stopping them – for you cannot stop them till you understand them – you are told that these modes of mind are fivefold in their nature. They are pentads. The Sutra, as usually translated, says "the Vrittis are five-fold (panchatayyah)," but pentad is a more accurate rendering of the word pancha-tayyah, in the original, than fivefold. The word pentad at once recalls to you the way in which the chemist speaks of a monad, triad, heptad, when he deals with elements. The elements with which the chemist is dealing are related to the unit-element in different ways. Some elements are related to it in one way only, and are called monads; others are related in two ways, and are called duads, and so on.

Is this applicable to the states of mind also? Recall the shloka of the Bhagavad-Gita in which it is said that the Jiva goes out into the world, drawing round him the five senses and mind as sixth. That may throw a little light on the subject. You have five senses, the five ways of knowing, the five jnanendriyas or organs of knowing. Only by these five senses can you know the outer world. Western psychology says that nothing exists in thought that does not exist in sensation. That is not true universally; it is not true of the abstract mind, nor wholly of the concrete. But there is a great deal of truth in it. Every idea is a pentad. It is made up of five elements. Each element making up the idea comes from one of the senses, and of these there are at present five. Later on every idea will be a heptad, made up of seven elements. For the present, each has five qualities, which build up the idea. The mind unites the whole together into a single thought, synthesises the five sensations. If you think of an orange and analyse your thought of an orange, you will find in it: colour, which comes through the eye; fragrance, which comes through the nose; taste, which comes through the tongue; roughness or smoothness, which comes through the sense of touch; and you would hear musical notes made by the vibrations of the molecules, coming through the sense of hearing, were it keener. If you had a perfect sense of hearing you would hear the sound of the orange also, for wherever there is vibration there is sound. All this, synthesised by the mind into one idea, is an orange. That is the root reason for the "association of ideas". It is not only that a fragrance recalls the scene and the circumstances under which the fragrance was observed, but because every impression is made through all the five senses and, therefore, when one is stimulated, the others are recalled. The mind is like a prism. If you put a prism in the path of a ray of white light, it will break it up into its seven constituent rays and seven colours will appear. Put another prism in the path of these seven rays, and as they pass through the prism, the process is reversed and the seven become one white light. The mind is like the second prism. It takes in the five sensations that enter through the senses, and combines them into a single precept. As at the present stage of evolution the senses are five only, it unites the five sensations into one idea. What the white ray is to the seven- coloured light, that a thought or idea is to the fivefold sensation. That is the meaning of the much controverted Sutra: "Vrittayah-panchatayych," "the vrittis, or modes of the mind, are pentads." If you look at it in that way, the later teachings will be more clearly understood.

As I have already said, that sentence, that nothing exists in thought which is not in sensation, is not the whole truth. Manas, the sixth sense, adds to the sensations its own pure elemental nature. What is that nature that you find thus added? It is the establishment of a relation, that is really what the mind adds. All thinking is the "establishment of relations," and the more closely you look into that phrase, the more you will realise how it covers all the varied processes of the mind. The very first process of the mind is to become aware of an outside world. However dimly at first, we become aware of something outside ourselves – a process generally called perception. I use the more general term "establishing a relation," because that runs through the whole of the mental processes, whereas perception is only a single thing. To use a well-known simile, when a little baby feels a pin pricking it, it is conscious of pain, but not at first conscious of the pin, nor yet conscious of where exactly the pin is. It does not recognise the part of the body in which the pin is. There is no perception, for perception is defined as relating a sensation to the object which causes the sensation. You only, technically speaking, "perceive" when you make a relation between the object and yourself. That is the very first of these mental processes, following on the heels of sensation. Of course, from the Eastern standpoint, sensation is a mental function also, for the senses are part of the cognitive faculty, but they are unfortunately classed with feelings in Western psychology. Now having established that relation between yourself and objects outside, what is the next process of the mind? Reasoning: that is, the establishing of relations between different objects, as perception is the establishment of your relation with a single object. When you have perceived many objects, then you begin to reason in order to establish relations between them. Reasoning is the establishment of a new relation, which comes out from the comparison of the different objects that by perception you have established in relation with yourself, and the result is a concept. This one phrase, "establishment of relations," is true all round. The whole process of thinking is the establishment of relations, and it is natural that it should be so, because the Supreme Thinker, by establishing a relation, brought matter into existence. Just as He, by establishing that primary relation between Himself and the Not-Self, makes a universe possible, so do we reflect His powers in ourselves, thinking by the same method, establishing relations, and thus carrying out every intellectual process.

Pleasure and Pain

Let us pass again from that to another statement made by this great teacher of Yoga: "Pentads are of two kinds, painful and non-painful." Why did he not say: "painful and pleasant"? Because he was an accurate thinker, a logical thinker, and he uses the logical division that includes the whole universe of discourse, A and Not-A, painful and non-painful. There has been much controversy among psychologists as to a third kind – indifferent. Some psychologists divide all feelings into three: painful, pleasant and indifferent. Feelings cannot be divided merely into pain and pleasure, there is a third class, called indifference, which is neither painful nor pleasant. Other psychologists say that indifference is merely pain or pleasure that is not marked enough to be called the one or the other. Now this controversy and tangle into which psychologists have fallen might be avoided if the primary division of feelings were a logical division. A and Not-A – that is the only true and logical division. Patanjali is absolutely logical and right. In order to avoid the quicksand into which the modern psychologists have fallen, he divides all vrittis, modes of mind, into painful and non-painful.

There is, however, a psychological reason why we should say "pleasure and pain," although it is not a logical division. The reason why there should be that classification is that the word pleasure and the word pain express two fundamental states of difference, not in the Self, but in the vehicles in which that Self dwells. The Self, being by nature unlimited, is ever pressing, so to say, against any boundaries which seek to limit him. When these limitations give way a little before the constant pressure of the Self, we feel "pleasure," and when they resist or contract, we feel "pain". They are not states of the Self so much as states of the vehicles, and states of certain changes in consciousness. Pleasure and pain belong to the Self as a whole, and not to any aspect of the Self separately taken. When pleasure and pain are marked off as belonging only to the desire nature, the objection arises: "Well, but in the exercise of the cognitive faculty there is an intense pleasure. When you use the creative faculty of the mind you are conscious of a profound joy in its exercise, and yet that creative faculty can by no means be classed with desire." The answer is: "Pleasure belongs to the Self as a whole. Where the vehicles yield themselves to the Self, and permit it to 'expand' as is its eternal nature, then what is called pleasure is felt." It has been rightly said: "Pleasure is a sense of moreness." Every time you feel pleasure, you will find the word "moreness" covers the case. It will cover the lowest condition of pleasure, the pleasure of eating. You are becoming more by appropriating to yourself a part of the Not-Self, food. You will find it true of the highest condition of bliss, union with the Supreme. You become more by expanding yourself to His infinity. When you have a phrase that can be applied to the lowest and highest with which you are dealing, you may be fairly sure it is all-inclusive, and that, therefore, "pleasure is moreness" is a true statement. Similarly, pain is "lessness".

If you understand these things your philosophy of life will become more practical, and you will be able to help more effectively people who fall into evil ways. Take drink. The real attraction of drinking lies in the fact that, in the first stages of it, a more keen and vivid life is felt. That stage is overstepped in the case of the man who gets drunk, and then the attraction ceases. The attraction lies in the first stages, and many people have experienced that, who would never dream of becoming drunk. Watch people who are taking wine and see how much more lively and talkative they become. There lies the attraction, the danger.

The real attraction in most coarse forms of excess is that they give an added sense of life, and you will never be able to redeem a man from his excess unless you know why he does it. Understanding the attractiveness of the first step, the increase of life, then you will be able to put your finger on the point of temptation, and meet that in your argument with him. So that this sort of mental analysis is not only interesting, but practically useful to every helper of mankind. The more you know, the greater is your power to help.

The next question that arises is: "Why does he not divide all feelings into pleasurable and not-pleasurable, rather than into 'painful and not-painful'?" A Westerner will not be at a loss to answer that: "Oh, the Hindu is naturally so very pessimistic, that he naturally ignores pleasure and speaks of painful and not-painful. The universe is full of pain." But that would not be a true answer. In the first place the Hindu is not pessimistic. He is the most optimistic of men. He has not got one solitary school of philosophy that does not put in its foreground that the object of all philosophy is to put an end to pain. But he is profoundly reasonable. He knows that we need not go about seeking happiness. It is already ours, for it is the essence of our own nature. Do not the Upanishads say: "The Self is bliss"? Happiness exists perennially within you. It is your normal state. You have not to seek it. You will necessarily be happy if you get rid of the obstacles called pain, which are in the modes of mind. Happiness is not a secondary thing, but pain is, and these painful things are obstacles to be got rid of. When they are stopped, you must be happy. Therefore Patanjali says: "The vrittis are painful and non-painful." Pain is an excrescence. It is a transitory thing. The Self, who is bliss, being the all-permeating life of the universe, pain has no permanent place in it. Such is the Hindu position, the most optimistic in the world.

Let us pause for a moment to ask: "Why should there be pain at all if the Self is bliss?" Just because the nature of the Self is bliss. It would be impossible to make the Self turn outward, come into manifestation, if only streams of bliss flowed in on him. He would have remained unconscious of the streams. To the infinity of bliss nothing could be added. If you had a stream of water flowing unimpeded in its course, pouring more water into it would cause no ruffling, the stream would go on heedless of the addition. But put an obstacle in the way, so that the free flow is checked, and the stream will struggle and fume against the obstacle, and make every endeavour to sweep it away. That which is contrary to it, that which will check its current's smooth flow, that alone will cause effort. That is the first function of pain. It is the only thing that can rouse the Self. It is the only thing that can awaken his attention. When that peaceful, happy, dreaming, in turned Self finds the surge of pain beating against him, he awakens: "What is this, contrary to my nature, antagonistic and repulsive, what is this?" It arouses him to the fact of a surrounding universe, an outer world. Hence in psychology, in yoga, always basing itself on the ultimate analysis of the fact of nature, pain is the thing that asserts itself as the most important factor in Self-realisation; that which is other than the Self will best spur the Self into activity. Therefore we find our commentator, when dealing with pain, declares that the karmic receptacle the causal body, that in which all the seeds of karma are gathered Up, has for its builder all painful experiences; and along that line of thought we come to the great generalisation: the first function of pain in the universe is to arouse the Self to turn himself to the outer world, to evoke his aspect of activity.

The next function of pain is the organisation of the vehicles. Pain makes the man exert himself, and by that exertion the matter of his vehicles gradually becomes organised. If you want to develop and organise your muscles, you make efforts, you exercise them, and thus more life flows into them and they become strong. Pain is necessary that the Self may force his vehicles into making efforts which develop and organise them. Thus pain not only awakens awareness, it also organises the vehicles.

It has a third function also. Pain purifies. We try to get rid of that which causes us pain. It is contrary to our nature, and we endeavour to throw it away. All that is against the blissful nature of the Self is shaken by pain out of the vehicles; slowly they become purified by suffering, and in that way become ready for the handling of the Self.

It has a fourth function. Pain teaches. All the best lessons of life come from pain rather than from joy. When one is becoming old, as I am and I look on the long life behind me, a life of storm and stress, of difficulties and efforts, I see something of the great lessons pain can teach. Out of my life story could efface without regret everything that it has had of joy and happiness, but not one pain would I let go, for pain is the teacher of wisdom.

It has a fifth function. Pain gives power. Edward Carpenter said, in his splendid poem of "Time and Satan," after he had described the wrestling's and the overthrows: 'Every pain that I suffered in one body became a power which I wielded in the next." Power is pain transmuted.

Hence the wise man, knowing these things, does not shrink from pain; it means purification, wisdom, power.

It is true that a man may suffer so much pain that for this incarnation he may be numbed by it, rendered wholly or partially useless. Especially is this the case when the pain has deluged in childhood. But even then, he shall reap his harvest of good later. By his past, he may have rendered present pain inevitable, but none the less can he turn it into a golden opportunity by knowing and utilising its functions.

You may say: "What use then of pleasure, if pain is so splendid a thing?" From pleasure comes illumination. Pleasure enables the Self to manifest. In pleasure all the vehicles of the Self are made harrnonious; they all vibrate together; the vibrations are rhythmical, not jangled as they are in pain, and those rhythmical vibrations permit that expansion of the Self of which I spoke, and thus lead up to illumination, the knowledge of the Self. And if that be true, as it is true, you will see that pleasure plays an immense part in nature, being of the nature of the Self, belonging to him. When it harmonises the vehicles of the Self from outside, it enables the Self more readily to manifest himself through the lower selves within us. Hence happiness is a condition of illumination. That is the explanation of the value of the rapture of the mystic; it is an intense joy. A tremendous wave of bliss, born of love triumphant, sweeps over the whole of his being, and when that great wave of bliss sweeps over him, it harmonises the whole of his vehicles, subtle and gross alike, and the glory of the Self is made manifest and he sees the face of his God. Then comes the wonderful illumination, which for the time makes him unconscious of all the lower worlds. It is because for a moment the Self is realising himself as divine, that it is possible for him to see that divinity which is cognate to himself. So you should not fear joy any more than you fear pain, as some unwise people do, dwarfed by a mistaken religionism. That foolish thought which you often find in an ignorant religion, that pleasure is rather to be dreaded, as though God grudged joy to His children, is one of the nightmares born of ignorance and terror. The Father of life is bliss. He who is joy cannot grudge Himself to His children, and every reflection of joy in the world is a reflection of the Divine Life, and a manifestation of the Self in the midst of matter. Hence pleasure has its function as well as pain and that also is welcome to the wise, for he understands and utilises it. You can easily see how along this line pleasure and pain become equally welcome. Identified with neither, the wise man takes either as it comes, knowing its purpose. When we understand the places of joy and of pain, then both lose their power to bind or to upset us. If pain comes, we take it and utilise it. If joy comes, we take it and utilise it. So we may pass through life, welcoming both pleasure and pain, content whichever may come to us, and not wishing for that which is for the moment absent. We use both as means to a desired end; and thus we may rise to a higher indifference than that of the stoic, to the true vairagya; both pleasure and pain are transcended, and the Self remains, who is bliss.

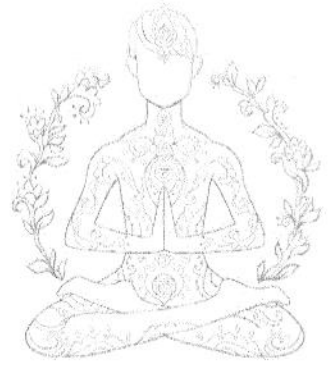

Lecture 4

Yoga as Practice

In dealing with the third section of the subject, I drew your attention to the states of mind, and pointed out to you that, according to the Sanskrit word vritti, those states of mind should be regarded as ways m which the mind exists, or, to use the philosophical phrase of the West, they are modes of mind, modes of mental existence. These are the states which are to be inhibited, put an end to, abolished, reduced into absolute quiescence. The reason for this inhibition is the production of a state which allows the higher mind to pour itself into the lower. To put it in another way: the lower mind, unruffled, waveless, reflects the higher, as a waveless lake reflects the stars. You will remember the phrase used in the Upanishad, which puts it less technically and scientifically, but more beautifully, and declares that in the quietude of the mind and the tranquility of the senses, a man may behold the majesty of the Self. The method of producing this quietude is what we have now to consider.

Inhibition of States of Mind

Two ways, and two ways only, there are of inhibiting these modes, these ways of existence, of the mind. They were given by Sri Krishna in the Bhagavad-Gita, when Arjuna complained that the mind was impetuous, strong, difficult to bend, hard to curb as the wind. His answer was definite: "Without doubt, O mighty-armed, the mind is hard to curb and restless; but it may be curbed by constant practice (abhyasa) and by dispassion (vai-ragya)."

These are the two methods, the only two methods, by which this restless, storm-tossed mind can be reduced to peace and quietude. Vai-ragya and abhyasa, they are the only two methods, but when steadily practiced they inevitably bring about the result.

Let us consider what these two familiar words imply. Vai-ragya, or dispassion, has as its main idea the clearing away of all passion for, attraction to, the objects of the senses, the bonds which are made by desire between man and the objects around him. Raga is "passion, addiction," that which binds a man to things. The prefix "vi" – changing to "vai" by a grammatical rule – means "without," or "in opposition to". Hence vai-ragya is "non-passion, absence of passion," not bound, tied or related to any of these outside objects. Remembering that thinking is the establishing of relations, we see that the getting rid of relations will impose on the mind the stillness that is Yoga. All raga must be entirely put aside. We must separate ourselves from it. We must acquire the opposite condition, where every passion is stilled, where no attraction for the objects of desire remains, where all the bonds that unite the man to surrounding objects are broken. "When the bonds of the heart are broken, then the man becomes immortal."

How shall this dispassion be brought about? There is only one right way of doing it. By slowly and gradually drawing ourselves away from outer objects through the more potent attraction of the Self. The Self is ever attracted to the Self. That attraction alone can turn these vehicles away from the alluring and repulsive objects that surround them; free from all raga, no more establishing relations with objects, the separated Self finds himself liberated and free, and union with the one Self becomes the sole object of desire. But not instantly, by one supreme effort, by one endeavour, can this great quality of dispassion become the characteristic of the man bent on Yoga. He must practice dispassion constantly and steadfastly. That is implied in the word joined with dispassion, abhyasa or practice. The practice must be constant, continual and unbroken. "Practice" does not mean only meditation, though this is the sense in which the word is generally used; it means the deliberate, unbroken carrying out of dispassion in the very midst of the objects that attract.

In order that you may acquire dispassion, you must practice it in the everyday things of life. I have said that many confine abhyasa to meditation. That is why so few people attain to Yoga. Another error is to wait for some big opportunity. People prepare themselves for some tremendous sacrifice and forget the little things of everyday life, in which the mind is knitted to objects by a myriad tiny threads. These things, by their pettiness, fail to attract attention, and in waiting for the large thing, which does not come, people lose the daily practice of dispassion towards the little things that are around them. By curbing desire at every moment, we become indifferent to all the objects that surround us. Then, when the great opportunity comes, we seize it while scarce aware that it is upon us. Every day, all day long, practice – that is what is demanded from the aspirant to Yoga, for only on that line can success come; and it is the wearisomeness of this strenuous, continued endeavour that tires out the majority of aspirants.

I must here warn you of a danger. There is a rough-and- ready way of quickly bringing about dispassion. Some say to you: "Kill out all love and affection; harden your hearts; become cold to all around you; desert your wife and children, your father and mother, and fly to the desert or the jungle; put a wall between yourself and all objects of desire; then dispassion will be yours." It is true that it is comparatively easy to acquire dispassion in that way. But by that you kill more than desire. You put round the Self, who is love, a barrier through which he is unable to pierce. You cramp yourself by encircling yourself with a thick shell, and you cannot break through it. You harden yourself where you ought to be softened; you isolate yourself where you ought to be embracing others; you kill love and not only desire, forgetting that love clings to the Self and seeks the Self, while desire clings to the sheaths of the Self, the bodies in which the Self is clothed. Love is the desire of the separated Self for union with all other separated Selves. Dispassion is the non-attraction to matter – a very different thing. You must guard love – for it is the very Self of the Self. In your anxiety to acquire dispassion do not kill out love. Love is the life in everyone of us, separated Selves. It draws every separated Self to the other Self. Each one of us is a part of one mighty whole. Efface desire as regards the vehicles that clothe the Self, but do not efface love as regards the Self, that never-dying force which draws Self to Self. In this great up-climbing, it is far better to suffer from love rather than to reject it, and to harden your hearts against all ties and claims of affection. Suffer for love, even though the suffering be bitter. Love, even though the love be an avenue of pain. The pain shall pass away, but the love shall continue to grow, and in the unity of the Self you shall finally discover that love is the great attracting force which makes all things one.

Many people, in trying to kill out love, only throw themselves back, becoming less human, not superhuman; by their mistaken attempts. It is by and through human ties of love and sympathy that the Self unfolds. It is said of the Masters that They love all humanity as a mother loves her firstborn son. Their love is not love watered down to coolness, but love for all raised to the heat of the highest particular loves of smaller souls. Always mistrust the teacher who tells you to kill out love, to be indifferent to human affections. That is the way which leads to the left-hand path.

Meditation with and without Seed

The next step is our method of meditation. What do we mean by meditation? Meditation cannot be the same for every man. Though the same in principle, namely, the steadying of the mind, the method must vary with the temperament of the practitioner. Suppose that you are a strong-minded and intelligent man, fond of reasoning. Suppose that connected links of thought and argument have been to you the only exorcise of the mind. Utilise that past training. Do not imagine that you can make your mind still by a single effort. Follow a logical chain of reasoning, step by step, link after link; do not allow the mind to swerve a hair's breadth from it. Do not allow the mind to go aside to other lines of thought. Keep it rigidly along a single line, and steadiness will gradually result. Then, when you have worked up to your highest point of reasoning and reached the last link of your chain of argument, and your mind will carry you no further, and beyond that you can see nothing, then stop. At that highest point of thinking, cling desperately to the last link of the chain, and there keep the mind poised, in steadiness and strenuous quiet, waiting for what may come. After a while, you will be able to maintain this attitude for a considerable time.

For one in whom imagination is stronger than the reasoning faculty, the method by devotion, rather than by reasoning, is the method. Let him call imagination to his help. He should picture some scene, in which the object of his devotion forms the central figure, building it up, bit by bit, as a painter paints a picture, putting in it gradually all the elements of the scene He must work at it as a painter works on his canvas, line by line, his brush the brush of imagination. At first the work will be very slow, but the picture soon begins to present itself at call. Over and over he should picture the scene, dwelling less and less on the surrounding objects and more and more on the central figure which is the object of his heart's devotion. The drawing of the mind to a point, in this way, brings it under control and steadies it, and thus gradually, by this use of the imagination he brings the mind under command. The object of devotion will be according to the man's religion. Suppose – as is the case with many of you – that his object of devotion is Sri Krishna; picture Him in any scene of His earthly life, as in the battle of Kurukshetra. Imagine the armies arrayed for battle on both sides; imagine Arjuna on the floor of the chariot, despondent, despairing; then come to Sri Krishna, the Charioteer, the Friend and Teacher. Then, fixing your mind on the central figure, let your heart go out to Him with one pointed devotion. Resting on Him, poise yourself in silence and, as before, wait for what may come.

This is what is called "meditation with seed". The central figure, or the last link in reasoning, that is "the seed". You have gradually made the vagrant mind steady by this process of slow and gradual curbing, and at last you are fixed on the central thought, or the central figure, and there you are poised. Now let even that go. Drop the central thought, the idea, the seed of meditation. Let everything go. But keep the mind in the position gained, the highest point reached, vigorous and alert. This is meditation without a seed. Remain poised, and wait in the silence and the void. You are in the "cloud," before described, and pass through the condition before sketched. Suddenly there will be a change, a change unmistakable, stupendous, incredible. In that silence, as said, a Voice shall be heard. In that void, a Form shall reveal itself. In that empty sky, a Sun shall rise, and in the light of that Sun you shall realise your own identity with it, and know that that which is empty to the eye of sense is full to the eye of Spirit, that that which is silence to the ear of sense is full of music to the ear of Spirit.

Along such lines you can learn to bring into control your mind, to discipline your vagrant thought, and thus to reach illumination. One word of warning. You cannot do this, while you are trying meditation with a seed. until you are able to cling to your seed definitely for a considerable time, and maintain throughout an alert attention. It is the emptiness of alert expectation. not the emptiness of impending sleep. If your mind be not in that condition, its mere emptiness is dangerous. It leads to medium ship, to possession, to obsession. You can wisely aim at emptiness, only when you have so disciplined the mind that it can hold for a considerable time to a single point and remain alert when that point is dropped.

The question is sometimes asked: "Suppose that I do this and succeed in becoming unconscious of the body; suppose that I do rise into a higher region; is it quite sure that I shall come back again to the body? Having left the body, shall I be certain to return?"

The idea of non-return makes a man nervous. Even if he says that matter is nothing and Spirit is everything, he yet does not like to lose touch with his body and, losing that touch, by sheer fear, he drops back to the earth after having taken so much trouble to leave it. You should, however, have no such fear. That which will draw you back again is the trace of your past, which remains under all these conditions.

The question is of the same kind as: "Why should a state of Pralaya ever come to an end, and a new state of Manvantara begin?" And the answer is the same from the Hindu psychological standpoint; because, although you have dropped the very seed of thought, you cannot destroy the traces which that thought has left, and that trace is a germ, and it tends to draw again to itself matter, that it may express itself once more. This trace is what is called the privation of matter – samskara. Far as you may soar beyond the concrete mind, that trace, left in the thinking principle, of what you have thought and have known, that remains and will inevitably draw you back. You cannot escape your past and, until your life-period is over, that samskara will bring you back. It is this also which, at the close of the heavenly life, brings a man back to rebirth. It is the expression of the law of rhythm. In Light on the Path, that wonderful occult treatise, this state is spoken of and the disciple is pictured as in the silence. The writer goes on to say: "Out of the silence that is peace a resonant voice shall arise. And this voice will say: 'It is not well; thou hast reaped, now thou must sow.' And knowing this voice to be the silence itself, thou wilt obey."

What is the meaning of that phrase: "Thou hast reaped, now thou must show?" It refers to the great law of rhythm which rules even the Logoi, the Ishvaras – the law of the Mighty Breath, the out-breathing and the in-breathing, which compels every fragment which is separated for a time. A Logos may leave His universe, and it may drop away when He turns His gaze inward, for it was He who gave reality to it.

He may plunge into the infinite depths of being, but even then there is the samskara of the past universe, the shadowy latent memory, the germ of maya from which He cannot escape. To escape from it would be to cease to be Ishvara, and to become Brahma Nirguna. There is no Ishvara without maya, there is no maya without Ishvara. Even in pralaya, a time comes when the rest is over and the inner life again demands manifestation; then the outward turning begins and a new universe comes forth. Such is the law of rest and activity: activity followed by rest; rest followed again by the desire for activity; and so the ceaseless wheel of the universe, as well as of human lives, goes on. For in the eternal, both rest and activity are ever present, and in that which we call Time, they follow each other, although in eternity they be simultaneous and ever-existing.

The Use of Mantras

Let us see how far we can help ourselves in this difficult work. I will draw your attention to one fact which is of enormous help to the beginner.

Your vehicles are ever restless. Every vibration in the vehicle produces a corresponding change in consciousness. Is there any way to check these vibrations, to steady the vehicle, so that consciousness may be still? One method is the repeating of a mantra. A mantra is a mechanical way of checking vibration. Instead of using the powers of the will and of imagination, you save these for other purposes, and use the mechanical resource of a mantra. A mantra is a definite succession of sounds. Those sounds, repeated rhythmically over and over again in succession, synchronise the vibrations of the vehicles into unity with themselves. Hence a mantra cannot be translated; translation alters the sounds. Not only in Hinduism, but in Buddhism, in Roman Catholicism, in Islam, and among the Parsis, mantras are found, and they are never translated, for when you have changed the succession and order of the sounds, the mantra ceases to be a mantra. If you translate the words, you may have a very beautiful prayer, but not a mantra. Your translation may be beautiful inspired poetry, but it is not a living mantra. It will no longer harmonise the vibrations of the surrounding sheaths, and thus enable the consciousness to become still. The poetry, the inspired prayer, these are mentally translatable. But a mantra is unique and untranslatable. Poetry is a great thing: it is often an inspirer of the soul, it gives gratification to the ear, and it may be sublime and beautiful, but it is not a mantra.

Attention

Let us consider concentration. You ask a man if he can concentrate. He at once says: "Oh! it is very difficult. I have often tried and failed." But put the same question in a different way, and ask him: "Can you pay attention to a thing?" He will at once say: "Yes, I can do that."

Concentration is attention. The fixed attitude of attention, that is concentration. If you pay attention to what you do, your mind will be concentrated. Many sit down for meditation and wonder why they do not succeed. How can you suppose that half an hour of meditation and twenty- three and a half hours of scattering of thought throughout the day and night, will enable you to concentrate during the half hour? You have undone during the day and night what you did in the morning, as Penelope unravelled the web she wove. To become a Yogi, you must be attentive all the time. You must practice concentration every hour of your active life. Now you scatter your thoughts for many hours, and you wonder that you do not succeed. The wonder would be if you did. You must pay attention every day to everything you do. That is, no doubt, hard to do, and you may make it easier in the first stages by choosing out of your day's work a portion only, and doing that portion with perfect, unflagging attention. Do not let your mind wander from the thing before you. It does not matter what the thing is. It may be the adding up of a column of figures, or the reading of a book. Anything will do. It is the attitude of the mind that is important and not the object before it. This is the only way of learning concentration. Fix your mind rigidly on the work before you for the time being, and when you have done with it, drop it. Practise steadily in this way for a few months, and you will be surprised to find how easy it becomes to concentrate the mind. Moreover, the body will soon learn to do many things automatically. If you force it to do a thing regularly, it will begin to do it, after a time, of its own accord, and then you find that you can manage to do two or three things at the same time. In England, for instance, women are very fond of knitting. When a girl first learns to knit, she is obliged to be very intent on her fingers. Her attention must not wander from her fingers for a moment, or she will make a mistake. She goes on doing that day after day, and presently her fingers have learnt to pay attention to the work without her supervision, and they may be left to do the knitting while she employs the conscious mind on something else. It is further possible to train your mind as the girl has trained her fingers. The mind also, the mental body, can be so trained as to do a thing automatically. At last, your highest consciousness can always remain fixed on the Supreme, while the lower consciousness in the body will do the things of the body, and do them perfectly, because perfectly trained. These are practical lessons of Yoga.

Practice of this sort builds up the qualities you want, and you become stronger and better, and fit to go on to the definite study of Yoga.

Obstacles to Yoga

Before considering the capacities needed for this definite practice, let us run over the obstacles to Yoga as laid down by Patanjali.

The obstacles to Yoga are very inclusive. First, disease: if you are diseased you cannot practice Yoga; it demands sound health, for the physical strain entailed by it is great. Then languor of mind: you must be alert, energetic, in your thought. Then doubt: you must have decision of will, must be able to make up your mind. Then carelessness: this is one of the greatest difficulties with beginners; they read a thing carelessly, they are inaccurate. Sloth: a lazy man cannot be a Yogi; one who is inert, who lacks the power and the will to exert himself; how shall he make the desperate exertions wanted along this line? The next, worldly-mindedness, is obviously an obstacle. Mistaken ideas is another great obstacle, thinking wrongly about things. One of the great qualifications for Yoga is "right notion" "Right notion" means that the thought shall correspond with the outside truth; that a man shall he fundamentally true, so that his thought corresponds to fact; unless there is truth in a man, Yoga is for him impossible. Missing the point, illogical, stupid, making the important, unimportant and vice versa. Lastly, instability: which makes Yoga impossible, and even a small amount of which makes Yoga futile; the unstable man cannot be a yogi.

Capacities of Yoga

Can everybody practise Yoga? No. But every well-educated person can prepare for its future practice. For rapid progress you must have special capacities, as for anything else. In any of the sciences a man may study without being the possessor of very special capacity, although he cannot attain eminence therein; and so it is with Yoga. Anybody with a fair intelligence may learn something from Yoga which he may advantageously practice, but he cannot hope unless he starts with certain capacities, to be a success in Yoga in this life. It is only right to say that; for if any special science needs particular capacities in order to attain eminence therein, the science of sciences certainly cannot fall behind the ordinary sciences in the demands that it makes on its students.

Suppose I am asked: "Can I become a great mathematician?" What must be my answer? "You must have a natural aptitude and capacity for mathematics to be a great mathematician. If you have not that capacity, you cannot be a great mathematician in this life." But this does not mean that you cannot learn any mathematics. To be a great mathematician you must be born with a special capacity for mathematics. To be born with such a special capacity means that you have practiced it in very many lives and now you are born with it ready-made. It is the same with Yoga. Every man can learn a little of it. But to be a great Yogi means lives of practice. If these are behind you, you will have been born with the necessary faculties in the present birth.

There are three faculties which one must have to obtain success in Yoga. The first is a strong desire. "Desire ardently." Such a desire is needed to break the strong links of desire which knit you to the outer world. Moreover, without that strong desire you will never go through all the difficulties that bat your way.

You must have the conviction that you will ultimately succeed, and the resolution to go on until you do succeed. It must be a desire so ardent and so firmly rooted, that obstacles only make it more keen. To such a man an obstacle is like fuel that you throw on a fire. It burns but the more strongly as it catches hold of it and finds it fuel for the burning. So difficulties and obstacles are but fuel to feed the fire of the yogi's resolute desire. He only becomes the more firmly fixed, because he finds the difficulties.

If you have not this strong desire, its absence shows that you are new to the work, but you can begin to prepare for it in this life. You can create desire by thought; you cannot create desire by desire. Out of the desire nature, the training of the desire nature cannot come.

What is it in us that calls out desire? Look into your own mind, and you will find that memory and imagination are the two things that evoke desire most strongly. Hence thought is the means whereby all the changes in desire can be brought about. Thought, imagination, is the only creative power in you, and by imagination your powers are to be unfolded. The more you think of a desirable object, the stronger becomes the desire for it. Then think of Yoga as desirable, if you want to desire Yoga. Think about the results of Yoga and what it means for the world when you have become a yogi, and you will find your desire becoming stronger and stronger. For it is only by thought that you can manage desire. You can do nothing with it by itself. You want the thing, or you do not want it, and within the limits of the desire nature you are helpless in its grasp. As just said, you cannot change desire by desire. You must go into another region of your being, the region of thought, and by thought you can make yourself desire or not desire, exactly as you like, if only you will use the right means, and those means, after all, are fairly simple.

Why is it you desire to possess a thing? Because you think it will make you happier. But suppose you know by past experience that in the long run it does not make you happier, but brings you sorrow, trouble, distress. You have at once, ready to your hands, the way to get rid of that desire. Think of the ultimate results. Let your mind dwell carefully on all the painful things. Jump over the momentary pleasure, and fix your thought steadily on the pain which follows the gratification of that desire. And when you have done that for a month or so, the very sight of those objects of desire will repel you. You will have associated it in your mind with suffering, and will recoil from it instinctively. You will not want it. You have changed the want, and have changed it by your power of imagination. There is no more effective way of destroying a vice than by deliberately picturing the ultimate results of its indulgence. Persuade a young man who is inclined to be profligate to keep in his mind the image of an old profligate; show him the profligate worn out, desiring without the power to gratify; and if you can get him to think in that way, unconsciously he will begin to shrink from that which before attracted him; the very hideousness of the results frightens away the man from clinging to the object of desire. And the would-be yogi has to use his thought to mark out the desires he will permit, and the desires that he is determined to slay.

The next thing after a strong desire is a strong will. Will is desire transmuted, its directing is changed from without to within. If your will is weak, you must strengthen it. Deal with it as you do with other weak things: strengthen it by practice. If a boy knows that he has weak arms, he says: "My arms are weak, but I shall practice gymnastics, work on the parallel bars: thus my arms. will grow strong." It is the same with the will. Practice will make strong the little, weak will that you have at present.

Resolve, for example, saying: "I will do such and such thing every morning," and do it. One thing at a time is enough for a feeble will. Make yourself a promise to do such and such a thing at such a time, and you will soon find that you will be ashamed to break your promise. When you have kept such a promise to yourself for a day, make it for a week, then for a fortnight. Having succeeded, you can choose a harder thing to do, and so on. By this forcing of action, you strengthen the will. Day after day it grows greater in power, and you find your inner strength increases. First have a strong desire. Then transmute it into a strong will.

The third requisite for Yoga is a keen and broad intelligence. You cannot control your mind, unless you have a mind to control. Therefore you must develop your mind. You must study. By study, I do not mean the reading of books. I mean thinking. You may read a dozen books and your mind may be as feeble as in the beginning. But if you have read one serious book properly, then, by slow reading and much thinking, your intelligence will be nurtured and your; mind grow strong.

These are the things you want – a strong desire, an indomitable will, a keen intelligence. Those are the capacities that you must unfold in order that the practice of Yoga may be possible to you. If your mind is very unsteady, if it is a butterfly mind like a child's, you must make it steady. That comes by close study and thinking. You must unfold the mind by which you are to work.

Forth-going and Returning

It will help you, in doing this and in changing your desire, if you realise that the great evolution of humanity goes on along two paths – the Path of Forth-going, and the Path of Return.

On the Path, or marga, of Pravritti – forth-going on which are the vast majority of human beings, desires are necessary and useful. On that path, the more desire a man has, the better for his evolution. They are the motives that prompt to activity. Without these the stagnates, he is inert. Why should Isvara have filled the worlds with desirable objects if He did not intend that desire should be an ingredient in evolution? He deals with humanity as a sensible mother deals -with her child. She does not give lectures to the child on the advantages of walking nor explain to it learnedly the mechanism of the muscles of the leg. She holds a bright glittering toy before the child, and says: "Come and get it." Desire awakens, and the child begins to crawl, and so it learns to walk. So Isvara has put toys around us, but always just out of our reach, and He says: "Come, children, take these. Here are love, money, fame, social consideration; come and get them. Walk, make efforts for them." And we, like children, make great efforts and struggle along to snatch these toys. When we seize the toy, it breaks into pieces and is of no use. People fight and struggle and toil for wealth, and, when they become multi-millionaires, they ask: "How shall we spend this wealth?" I read of a millionaire in America, who was walking on foot from city to city, in order to distribute the vast wealth which he accumulated. He learned his lesson. Never in another life will that man be induced to put forth efforts for the toy of wealth. Love of fame, love of power, stimulate men to most strenuous effort. But when they are grasped and held in the hand, weariness is the result. The mighty statesman, the leader of the nation, the man idolised by millions – follow him home, and there you will see the weariness of power, the satiety that cloys passion. Does then God mock us with all the objects? No. The object has been to bring out the power of the Self to develop the capacity latent in man, and in the development of human faculty, the result of the great Lila may be seen. That is the way in which we learn to unfold the God within us; that is the result of the play of the divine Father with His children.

But sometimes the desire for objects is lost too early, and the lesson is but half learned. That is one of the difficulties in the India of today. You have a mighty spiritual philosophy, which was the natural expression for the souls who were born centuries ago. They were ready to throw away the fruit of action and to work for the Supreme to carry out His Will.

But the lesson for India at the present time is to wake up the desire. It may look like going back, but it is really a going forward. The philosophy is true, but it belonged to those older souls who were ready for it, and the younger souls now being born into the people are not ready for that philosophy. They repeat it by rote, they are hypnotised by it, and they sink down into inertia, because there is nothing they desire enough to force them to exertion. The consequence is that the nation as a whole is going downhill. The old lesson of putting different objects before souls of different ages, is forgotten, and everyone is now nominally aiming at ideal perfection, which can only be reached when the preliminary steps have been successfully mounted. It is the same as with the "Sermon on the Mount" in Christian countries, but there the practical common sense of the people bows to it and – ignores it. No nation tries to live by the "Sermon on the Mount" It is not meant for ordinary men and women, but for the saint. For all those who are on the Path of Forth-going, desire is necessary for progress.

What is the Path of Nivritti? It is the Path of Return. Their desire must cease; and the Self-determined will must take its place. The last object of desire in a person commencing the Path of Return is the desire to work with the Will of the Supreme; he harmonises his will with the Supreme Will, renounces all separate desires, and thus works to turn the wheel of life as long as such turning is needed by the law of Life. Desire on the Path of Forth-going becomes will on the Path of Return; the soul, in harmony with the Divine, works with the law. Thought on the Path of Forth-going is ever alert, flighty and changing; it becomes reason on the Path of Return; the yoke of reason is placed on the neck of the lower mind, and reason guides the bull. Work, activity, on the Path of Forth-going, is restless action by which the ordinary man is bound; on the Path of Return work becomes sacrifice, and thus its binding force is broken. These are, then, the manifestations of three aspects, as shown on the Paths of Forth-going and Return.

Bliss manifested as desire is changed into will
Wisdom manifested as thought is changed into reason.
Activity manifested as work is changed into sacrifice.

People very often ask with regard to this: "Why is will placed in the human being as the correspondence of bliss in the Divine?" The three great Divine qualities are: chit or consciousness; ananda or bliss; sat or existence. Now it is quite clear that the consciousness is reflected in intelligence in man – the same quality, only in miniature. It is equally clear that existence and activity belong to each other. You can only exist as you act outwards. The very form of the word shows It—"ex, out of"; it is manifested life. That leaves the third, bliss, to correspond with will, and some people are rather puzzled with that, and they ask: "What is the correspondence between bliss and will?" But if you come down to desire, and the objects of desire, you will be able to solve the riddle. The nature of the Self is bliss. Throw that nature down into matter and what will be the expression of the bliss nature? Desire for happiness, the seeking after desirable objects, which it imagines will give it the happiness which is of its own essential nature, and which it is continually seeking to realise amid the obstacles of the world. Its nature being bliss, it seeks for happiness and that desire for happiness is to be transmuted into will. All these correspondences have a profound meaning if you will only look into them, and that universal "will-to-live" translates itself as the "desire for happiness" that you find in every man and woman, in every sentient creature. Has it ever struck you how surely you are justifying that analysis of your own nature by the way you accept happiness as your right, and resent misery, and ask what you have done to deserve it? You do not ask the same about happiness, which is the natural result of your own nature. The thing that has to be explained is not happiness but pain, the things that are against the nature of the Self that is bliss. And so, looking into this, we see how desire and will are both the determination to be happy. But the one is ignorant, drawn out by outer objects; the other is self-conscious, initiated and ruled from within. Desire is evoked and directed from outside; and when the same aspect rules from within, it is will. There is no difference in their nature. Hence desire on the Path of Forth-going becomes will on the Path of Return.

When desire, thought and work are changed into will, reason and sacrifice, then the man is turning homewards, then he lives by renunciation.

When a man has really renounced, a strange change takes place. On the Path of Forth-going, you must fight for everything you want to get; on the Path of Return, nature pours her treasures at your feet. When a man has ceased to desire them, then all treasures pour down upon him, for he has become a channel through which all good gifts flow to those around him. Seek the good, give up grasping, and then everything will be yours. Cease to ask that your own little water tank may be filled, and you will become a pipe, joined to the living source of all waters, the source which never runs dry, the waters which spring up unfailingly. Renunciation means the power of unceasing work for the good of all, work which cannot fail, because wrought by the Supreme Worker through His servant.

If you are engaged in any true work of charity, and your means are limited and the wealth does not flow into your hands, what does it mean? It means that you have not yet learnt the true renunciation. You are clinging to the visible, to the fruit of action, and so the wealth does not pour through your hands.

Purification of Bodies

The unfolding of powers belongs to the side of consciousness; purification of bodies belongs to the side of matter. You must purify each of your three working bodies – mental, astral and physical. Without that purification you had better leave yoga alone. First of all, how shall you purify the thought body? By right thinking. Then you must use imagination, your great creative tool, once more. Imagine things, and, imagining them, you will form your thought-body into the organisation that you desire. Imagine something strongly, as the painter imagines when he is going to paint. Visualise an object if you have the power of visualisation at all: if you have not, try to make it. It is an artistic faculty, of course, hut most people have it more or less. See how far you can reproduce perfectly a face you see daily. By such practice you will be strengthening your imagination, and by strengthening your imagination you will be making the great tool with which you have to practice in Yoga.

There is another use of the imagination which is very valuable. If you will imagine in your thought-body the presence of the qualities that you desire to have, and the absence of those which you desire not to have, you are half-way to having and not having them. Also, many of the troubles of your life might be weakened if you would imagine them on right lines before you have to go through them. Why do you wait helplessly until you meet them in the physical world. If you thought of your coming trouble in the morning, and thought of yourself as acting perfectly in the midst of it (you should never scruple to imagine yourself perfect), when the thing turned up in the day, it would have lost its power, and you would no longer feel the sting to the same extent. Now each of you must have in your life something that troubles you. Think of yourself as facing that trouble and not minding it, and when it comes, you will be what you have been thinking. You might get rid of half your troubles and your faults, if you would deal with them through your imagination.

As the thought body, becomes purified in this way, you must turn to the astral body. The astral body is purified by right desire. Desire nobly, and the astral body will evolve the organs of good desires instead of the organs of evil ones. The secret of all progress is to think and desire the highest, never dwelling on the fault, the weakness, the error, but always on the perfected power, and slowly in that way you will be able to build up perfection in yourself. Think and desire, then, in order to purify the thought body and the astral body.

And how shall you purify the physical body? You must regulate it in all its activities – in sleep, in food, in exercise, in everything. You cannot have a pure physical body with impure mental and astral bodies so that the work of imagination helps also in the purification of the physical. But you must also regulate the physical body in all its activities. Take for instance, food. The Indian says truly that every sort of food has a dominant quality in it, either rhythm, or activity, or inertia, and that all foods fall under one of these heads. Now the man who is to be a yogi must not touch any food which is on the way to decay. Those things belong to the tamasic foods – all foods, for instance, of the nature of game, of venison, all food which is showing signs of decay (all alcohol is a product of decay), are to be avoided. Flesh foods come under the quality of activity. All flesh foods are really stimulants. All forms in the animal kingdom are built up to express animal desires and animal activities. The yogi cannot afford to use these in a body meant for the higher processes of thought. Vitality, yes, they will give that; strength, which does not last, they will give that; a sudden spurs of energy, yes, meat will give that; but those are not the things which the yogi wants; so he puts aside all those foods as not available for the work he desires, and chooses his food out of the most highly vitalised products. All the foods which tend to growth, those are the most highly vitalised, grain, out of which the new plant will grow, is packed full of the most nutritious substances; fruits; all those things which have growth as their next stage in the life cycle, those are the rhythmic foods, full of life, and building up a body sensitive and strong at the same time.

Dwellers on the Threshold

Of these there are many kinds. First, elementals. They try to bar the astral plane against man. And naturally so, because they are concerned with the building up of the lower kingdoms, these elementals of form, the Rupa Devas; and to them man is a really hateful creature, because of his destructive properties. That is why they dislike him so much. He spoils their work wherever he goes, tramples down vegetable things, and kills animals, so that the whole of that great kingdom of nature hates the name of man. They band themselves together to stop the one who is just taking his first conscious steps on the astral plane, and try to frighten him, for they fear that he is bringing destructiveness into the new world. They cannot do anything, if you do not mind them. When that rush of elemental force comes against the man entering on the astral plane, he must remain quiet, indifferent, taking up the position: "I am a higher product of evolution than you are; you can do nothing to me. I am your friend, not your enemy, Peace!" If he be strong enough to take up that position, the great wave of elemental force will roll aside and let him through. The seemingly causeless fears which some feel at night are largely due to this hostility. You are, at night, more sensitive to the astral plane than during the day, and the dislike of the beings on the plane for man is felt more strongly. But when the elementals find you are not destructive, not an embodiment of ruin, they become as friendly to you as they were before hostile. That is the first form of the dweller on the threshold. Here again the importance of pure and rhythmic food comes in; because if you use meat and alcohol, you attract the lower elementals of the plane, those that take pleasure in the scent of blood and spirits, and they will inevitably prevent your seeing and understanding things clearly. They will surge round you, impress their thoughts upon you, force their impressions on your astral body, so that you may have a kind of shell of objectionable hangers-on to your aura, who will much obstruct you in your efforts to see and hear correctly. That is the chief reason why everyone who is teaching Yoga on the right-hand path absolutely forbids indulgence in meat and alcohol.

The second form of the dweller on the threshold is the thought forms of our own past. Those forms, growing out of the evil of lives that lie behind us, thought forms of wickedness of all kinds, those face us when we first come into touch with the astral plane, really belonging to us, but appearing as outside forms, as objects; and they try to scare back their creator. You can only conquer them by sternly repudiating them: "You are no longer mine; you belong to my past, and not to my present. I will give you none of my life." Thus you will gradually exhaust and finally annihilate them. This is perhaps one of the most painful difficulties that one has to face in treading the astral plane in consciousness for the first time. Of course, where a person has in any way been mixed up with objectionable thought forms of the stronger kind, such as those brought about by practicing black magic, there this particular form of the dweller will be much stronger and more dangerous, and often desperate is the struggle between the neophyte and these dwellers from his past backed up by the masters of the black side.

Now we come to one of the most terrible forms of the dwellers on the threshold. Suppose a case in which a man during the past has steadily identified himself with the lower part of his nature and has gone against the higher, paralysing himself, using higher powers for lower purposes, degrading his mind to be the mere slave of his lower desires. A curious change takes place in him. The life which belongs to the Ego in him is taken up by the physical body, and assimilated with the lower lives of which the body is composed. Instead of serving the purposes of the Spirit, it is dragged away for tile purposes of the lower, and becomes part of the animal life belonging to the lower bodies, so that the Ego and his higher bodies are weakened, and the animal life of the lower is strengthened. Now under those conditions, the Ego will sometimes become so disgusted with his vehicles that when death relieves him of the physical body he will cast the others quite aside. And even sometimes during physical life he will leave the desecrated temple. Now after death, in these cases, the man generally reincarnates very quickly; for, having torn himself away from his astral and mental bodies, he has no bodies with which to live in the astral and mental worlds, and he must quickly form new ones and come again to rebirth here. Under these conditions the old astral and mental bodies are not disintegrated when the new mental and astral bodies are formed and born into the world, and the affinity between the old and new, both having had the same owner, the same tenant, asserts itself, and the highly vitalised old astral and mental bodies will attach themselves to the new astral and mental bodies, and become the most terrible form of the dweller on the threshold.

These are the various forms which the dweller may assume, and all are spoken of in books dealing with these particular subjects, though I do not know that you will find anywhere in a single book a definite classification like the above. In addition to these there are, of course, the direct attacks of the Dark Brothers, taking up various forms and aspects, and the most common form they will take is the form of some virtue which is a little bit in excess in the yogi. The yogi is not attacked through his vices, but through his virtues; for a virtue in excess becomes a vice. It is the extremes which are ever the vices; the golden mean is the virtue. And thus, virtues become tempters in the difficult regions of the astral and mental worlds, and are utilised by the Brothers of the Shadow in order to entrap the unwary.

I am not here speaking of the four ordinary ordeals of the astral plane: the ordeals by earth, water, fire and air. Those are mere trifles, hardly worth considering when speaking of these more serious difficulties. Of course, you have to learn that you are entirely master of astral matter, that earth cannot crush you, nor water drown you, etc. Those are, so to speak, very easy lessons. Those who belong to a Masonic body will recognise these ordeals as parts of the language they are familiar with in their Masonic ritual.

There is one other danger also. You may injure yourself by repercussion. If on the astral plane you are threatened with danger which belongs to the physical, but are unwise enough to think it can injure you, it will injure your physical body. You may get a wound, or a bruise, and so on, out of astral experiences. I once made a fool of myself in this way. I was in a ship going down and, as I was busy there, I saw that the mast of the ship was going to fall and, in a moment's forgetfulness, thought: "That mast will fall on me" that momentary thought had its result, for when I came back to the body in the morning, I had a large physical bruise where the mast fell. That is a frequent phenomenon until you have corrected the fault of the mind, which thinks instinctively the things which it is accustomed to think down here.

One protection you can make for yourself as you become more sensitive. Be rigorously truthful in thought, in word, indeed. Every thought, every desire, takes form in the higher world. If you are careless of truth here, you are creating a whole host of terrifying and deluding forms. Think truth, speak truth, live truth, and then you shall be free from the illusions of the astral world.

Preparation for Yoga

People say that I put the ideal of discipleship so very high that nobody can hope to become a disciple. But I have not said that no one can become a disciple who does not reproduce the description that is given of the perfect disciple. One may. But we do it at our own peril. A man may be thoroughly capable along one line, but have a serious fault along another. The serious fault will not prevent him from becoming a disciple, but he must suffer for it. The initiate pays for his faults ten times the price he would have had to pay for them as a man of the world. That is why I have put the ideal so high. I have never said that a person must come utterly up to the ideal before becoming a disciple, but I have said that the risks of becoming a disciple without these qualifications are enormous. It is the duty of those who have seen the results of going through the gateway with faults in character, to point out that it is well to get rid of these faults first. Every fault you carry through the gateway with you becomes a dagger to stab you on the other side. Therefore it is well to purify yourself as much as you can, before you are sufficiently evolved on any line to have the right to say: "I will pass through that gateway." That is what I intended to be understood when I spoke of qualifications for discipleship. I have followed along the ancient road which lays down these qualifications which the disciple should bring with him; and if he comes without them, then the word of Jesus is true, that he will be beaten with many stripes; for a man can afford to do in the outer world with small result what will bring terrible results upon him when once he is treading the Path.

The End

What is to be the end of this long struggle? What is the goal of the upward climbing, the prize of the great battle? What does the yogi reach at last? He reaches unity. Sometimes I am not sure that large numbers of people, if they realised what unity means, would really desire to reach it. There are many "virtues" of your ordinary life which will drop entirely away from you when you reach unity. Many things you admire will be no longer helps but hindrances, when the sense of unity begins to dawn. All those qualities so useful in ordinary life – such as moral indignation, repulsion from evil, judgment of others – have no room where unity is realised. When you feel repulsion from evil, it is a sign that your Higher Self is beginning to awaken, is seeing the dangers of evil: he drags the body forcibly away from it. That is the beginning of the conscious moral life. Hatred of evil is better at that stage than indifference to evil. It is a necessary stage. But repulsion cannot be felt when a man has realised unity, when he sees God made manifest in man. A man who knows unity cannot judge another. "I judge no man," said the Christ. He cannot be repelled by anyone. The sinner is himself, and how shall he be repelled from himself? For him there is no "I" or "Thee," for we are one.

This is not a thing that many honestly wish for. It is not a thing that many honestly desire. The man who has realised unity knows no difference between himself and the vilest wretch that walks the earth. He sees only the God that walks in the sinner, and knows that the sin is not in the God but in the sheath. The difference is only there. He who has realised the inner greatness of the Self never pronounces judgment upon another, knows that other as himself, and he himself as that other – that is unity. We talk brotherhood, but how many of us really practice it? And even that is not the thing the yogi aims at. Greater than brotherhood are identity and realisation of the Self as one. The Sixth Root Race will carry brotherhood to the highest point. The Seventh Root Race will know identity, will realise the unity of the human race. To catch a glimpse of the beauty of that high conception, the greatness of the unity in which "I" and "mine," "you" and "yours" have vanished, in which we are all one life, even to do that lifts the whole nature towards divinity, and those who can even see that unity is fair; they are the nearer to the realisation of the Beauty that is God.

PAPERBACK NON-FICTION

- 12 Years A Slave by Solomon Northup, ISBN: 9789390492374
- 51 Must Know Facts About Albert Einstein by GP Editors, ISBN: 9789354991486
- 51 Must Know Facts About Brain by GP Editors, ISBN: 9789354994371
- A Theory of Human Motivation by Abraham H. Maslow, ISBN: 9789354993732
- Becoming a Writer by Dorothea Brande, ISBN: 9789389157093
- Believe in Yourself by Joseph Murphy, ISBN: 9789388118385
- Chanakya Neeti by Chanakya, ISBN: 9789389716276
- Children's Objective Quiz by Azeem Ahmad Khan, ISBN: 9788180320781
- Creative Mind and Success by Ernest Holmes, ISBN: 9789354994661
- Delighting in God by AW Tozer, ISBN: 9788194748632
- Feeling is the Secret by Neville Goddard, ISBN: 9789389157109
- Five Chimneys by Olga Lengyel, ISBN: 9789354991127
- Five Lessons by Neville Goddard, ISBN: 9789354991134
- Gravity by George Gamow, ISBN: 9789388118484
- Great Speeches of Abraham Lincoln, ISBN: 9789380914336
- How to Attract Money by Joseph Murphy, ISBN: 9789388118408
- How to Develop Self Confidence and... by Dale Carnegie, ISBN: 9789387669000
- How to Enjoy Your Life and Your Job by Dale Carnegie, ISBN: 9789387669017
- How to Own Your Own Mind by Napoleon Hill, ISBN: 9789354991189
- How to Stop Worrying and Start Living by Dale Carnegie, ISBN: 9789380914817
- How to Use the Power of Prayer by Joseph Murphy, ISBN: 9789354994395
- How to Win Friends and Influence People by Dale Carnegie, ISBN: 9788180320217
- If You Want to Write by Brenda Ueland, ISBN: 9789389716290
- Know Your Worth by NK Sondhi, ISBN: 9788180320231
- Life in Corona by NK Sondhi, ISBN: 9789354990571

Develop your reading habit | **Gift books to your friends**

PAPERBACK NON-FICTION

- Madhubala by Manju Gupta, ISBN: 9789380914961
- Mahatma Gandhi by Romain Rolland, ISBN: 9789354994456
- Meditation and Its Methods by Swami Vivekananda, ISBN: 9789389716320
- Meditations by Marcus Aurelius, ISBN: 9789388118736
- Mein Kampf by Adolf Hitler, ISBN: 9789380914855
- Memory by William Walker Atkinson, ISBN: 9789390492800
- My Inventions: An Autobiography by Nikola Tesla, ISBN: 9789388118132
- Quiz For All by Azeem Ahmad Khan, ISBN: 9788180320897
- State and Revolution by Vladimir Ilich Lenin, ISBN: 9789354990922
- Stolen Legacy by George J.M. James, ISBN: 9789354994494
- Success Through a Positi. Mental Attitude by Napoleon Hill, ISBN: 9789390492435
- Tao Te Ching by Lao Tzu, ISBN: 9788194764823
- The Alchemy of Happiness by Al-Ghazzali, ISBN: 9789387669505
- The Art of Living by Epictetus, ISBN: 9789354993817
- The Art of Public Speaking by Dale Carnegie, ISBN: 9788180320422
- The Autobiography of a Yogi by Paramahansa Yogananda, ISBN: 9789380914602
- The Complete Prophecies of Nostradamus by Nostradamus, ISBN: 9789354994234
- The Dhammapada by Gautama Buddha, ISBN: 9789390492817
- The Dynamic Laws of Prosperity by Catherine Ponder, ISBN: 9789388118156
- The Elements of Style by William Strunk, ISBN: 9789389157123
- The Federalist Papers by Alexander Hamilton, ISBN: 9789390492862
- The Interpretation of Dreams by Sigmund Freud, ISBN: 9789390492879
- The Knowledge of the Holy by AW Tozer, ISBN: 9789389157130
- The Kybalion: Philo. of Egypt & Greece by Three Initiates, ISBN: 9789354994579
- The Magic of Faith by Joseph Murphy, ISBN: 9789388118743

Develop your reading habit | **Gift books to your friends**

PAPERBACK NON-FICTION

- The Miracles of Your Mind by Joseph Murphy, ISBN: 9788180320743
- The Path of Prosperity by James Allen, ISBN: 9789387669512
- The Power of Concentration by Theron Q. Dumont, ISBN: 9789388118064
- The Power of the Spoken Word by Florence Scovel Shinn, ISBN: 9789390492893
- The Problem of Increasing Human Energy by Nikola Tesla, ISBN: 9789354990953
- The Problems of Philosophy by Bertrand Russell, ISBN: 9789354994296
- The Quick and Easy Way to Effec. Speaking by Dale Carnegie, ISBN: 9789387669031
- The Science of Being Great by Wallace D. Wattles, ISBN: 9789354993886
- The Science of Getting Rich by Wallace D. Wattles, ISBN: 9788180320972
- The Science of Mind by Ernest Holmes, ISBN: 9789354993909
- The Secret of Imagining by Neville Goddard, ISBN: 9789354991271
- The Secret Teachings of All Ages by Manly P. Hall, ISBN: 9789390492046
- The Seven Laws of Teaching by John Milton Gregory, ISBN: 9789387669413
- The Story of My Life by Helen Keller, ISBN: 9789380914541
- The Success System that Never Fails by W.C. Stone, ISBN: 9789390492114
- The Ultimate Guide To Success by Julia Seton, ISBN: 9789390492350
- The Wit and Wisdom of Gandhi by Mahatma Gandhi, ISBN: 9789380914039
- The Yoga Sutras of Patanjali by Patanjali, ISBN: 9789389716351
- Think and Grow Rich by Napoleon Hill, ISBN: 9788180320255
- Thought Vibration by William Walker Atkinson, ISBN: 9789389157154
- Thoughts are Things by Prentice Mulford, ISBN: 9789354994326
- Up From Slavery by Booker T. Washington, ISBN: 9789380914565
- Value, Price, and Profit by Karl Marx, ISBN: 9789354993978
- Wake Up and Live by Dorothea Brande, ISBN: 9789387669574
- Who were the Shudras by Dr. B.R. Ambedkar, ISBN: 9789354991028

Develop your reading habit | **Gift books to your friends**